D1309206

The assessment of
VISUAL FUNCTION

Edited by

ALBERT M. POTTS, M.D., Ph.D.

Professor of Ophthalmology,
Director of Research in Ophthalmology, University of Chicago,
Chicago, Illinois

With 149 illustrations

THE C. V. MOSBY COMPANY

Saint Louis   1972

Carl F. Shepard Memorial Library
Illinois College of Optometry   10338

Copyright © 1972 by The C. V. Mosby Company

All rights reserved. No part of this book may be reproduced
in any manner without written permission of the publisher.

Printed in the United States of America

International Standard Book Number 0-8016-4008-3

Library of Congress Catalog Card Number 71-190609

Distributed in Great Britain by Henry Kimpton, London

CONTRIBUTORS

MATHEW ALPERN, Ph.D.

Professor of Physiological Optics in Departments of Ophthalmology and Physiology;
Professor of Psychology in Department of Psychology, University of Michigan,
Ann Arbor, Michigan

HERMANN M. BURIAN, M.D.

Emeritus Professor of Ophthalmology, University of Iowa, Iowa City, Iowa;
Professor of Ophthalmology, University of North Carolina, Chapel Hill, North Carolina;
Clinical Professor of Ophthalmology, Duke University,
Durham, North Carolina

ARTHUR H. KEENEY, M.D.

Director, Wills Eye Hospital; Professor and Chairman, Department of Ophthalmology,
Temple University, Philadelphia, Pennsylvania

ALEX E. KRILL, M.D.

Professor of Ophthalmology, University of Chicago, Chicago, Illinois

MATTHEW NEWMAN, M.D.

Instructor in Clinical Ophthalmology, Washington University, St. Louis, Missouri

JOEL POKORNY, Ph.D.

Assistant Professor of Ophthalmology, University of Chicago, Chicago, Illinois

ALBERT M. POTTS, M.D., Ph.D.

Professor of Ophthalmology, Director of Research in Ophthalmology,
University of Chicago, Chicago, Illinois

MELVIN L. RUBIN, M.D.

Professor of Ophthalmology, University of Florida, Gainesville, Florida

VIVIANNE C. SMITH, Ph.D.

Research Associate in Ophthalmology (Assistant Professor), University of Chicago,
Chicago, Illinois

PREFACE

The American Committee on Optics and Visual Physiology is composed of members appointed by the American Academy of Ophthalmology and Otolaryngology, the American Ophthalmological Society, the American Medical Association, and the Association for Research in Vision and Ophthalmology. The Committee's function is to propose standards for activities involving vision, to advise the parent societies on these areas, and to further the progress of ophthalmology by maximum utilization of our knowledge in optics and visual physiology.

It was in this last context that Dr. Hermann Burian, the recently retired chairman, proposed that the committee renew its activity. It was decided that a course be offered at the Academy meeting that emphasized the connection between basic science and ophthalmology. It was most logical to make that connection in terms of day-to-day practice. A necessary requirement of every clinical eye examination is assessment of function in order to measure impairment of function by disease. Each of the methods used to evaluate function has a scientific basis. The in-depth understanding of this basis makes a more effective physician who will be able to grow with the profession. As new methods are made available this basic knowledge will allow him to select those that are scientifically valid and that suit his needs. For less used methods, such as measurement of adaptation or electrophysiological techniques, basic understanding will allow proper referral.

At the same time the course was decided upon, it was realized that unified text material with the emphasis desired was not available. For this reason the instructors in the course, each of whom had special competence in his subject area, was invited to submit a chapter. The object in each section was to present the underlying scientific principles and then to explain the clinical methods based on these principles. Indications for use follow naturally. In two sections, those on adaptation and color vision, the subject is sufficiently complex to warrant separate chapters on the basic aspects by specialists in the respective areas. The section on practical aspects of depth perception emphasizes a different situation. Although binocularity and stereopsis are measured with relative ease and the literature on these areas is massive, stereopsis has only a modest connection with depth perception. In many of the activities of modern life—driving a car, crossing a street, flying a plane—depth perception is vital and stereopsis is of minor importance. As Professor Burian points out in his chapter, there are no adequate clinical methods for testing these practical aspects of depth perception; they need to be developed. The section on electrophysiological methods is somewhat different again. None of these methods is a routine office procedure. Hence emphasis is on understanding indications and procedures rather than on performing them. The result of all of the above considerations is the present volume.

In addition to the contributors whose role is evident, I wish to express my thanks to Mrs. Edith Goldman, whose help has been constant.

Albert M. Potts

CONTENTS

I Introduction

CHAPTER 1

*Visual acuity**

MELVIN L. RUBIN

When most individuals meet the term "visual acuity," their initial reaction is to a brilliant flash of a big Snellen letter E bursting into consciousness. Why not? Is not "Snellen acuity" just about synonymous with "visual acuity?" Is it not the basis for a clinical test that assesses macular function? I hope that after review of this chapter, you will be aware that (1) *Snellen* acuity is only one of many acuities and is by no means all there is to this subject, and (2) testing *macular* function is only one aspect of any acuity test.

Some type of visual acuity determination is performed by every ophthalmology practitioner every working day on a large variety of patients. But more often than not, the fine points of what he is actually testing are little appreciated and even less understood.

When a visual acuity chart is presented to a patient, images of the letters on that chart are formed by spectacles and the optical components of the eye. These images are squeezed through openings, battered about by irregularities in the optical media, distorted by the irregular receiving plane, completely rearranged (topologically) in an array of interacting neural cells and transmission fibers, and finally distributed to diverse areas in the brain—the cortex, subcortical association areas, and so forth. When the "images" of the letter stimuli finally enter consciousness, something that "makes sense" has to be interpreted by the observer. Thus any acuity test screens for a defect *anywhere* along the visual pathway, up to the final interpretation of the retinal image. In other words, this test tests the functional integrity not only of the macula but of the entire visual and psychic function.

Now, in speaking of an acuity test, we postponed a definition of what *acuities* are. Note please that we mention acui*ties,* since there are many more than the familiar one that is called "Snellen resolution."

Acuities are a group of "psychophysical" relationships, that is, the relation between a stimulus and a response. Visual stimuli presented to an observer are usually classified as either intensities or extensities and come in various strengths. If we speak of a *threshold* stimulus—that is, that stimulus that is just barely

---

*Part of the material in this section is modified from Rubin, M. L.: Visual acuities. In Rubin, M. L., and Walls, G. L.: Fundamentals of visual science, Springfield, Ill., 1969, Charles C Thomas, Publisher.

strong enough to elicit a response—we have a measure of how responsive is the system tested. If that response happens to be to an *intensity* of something, the reciprocal of that intensity is called a sensitivity; if, on the other hand, the threshold response is to a stimulus of a minimum *extent* (length or angular measurement), the reciprocal is termed an *acuity*. An acuity is then the reciprocal of a threshold angular extent. What that angle is will be discussed shortly.

PSYCHOPHYSICAL RELATIONSHIPS

Some elaboration of the term "psychophysical" is in order, for most of the methods for assessment of visual function in this volume come under the category of psychophysics. A "psychophysical" relationship is a relationship between a sensation and the stimulus causing it. This is a very broad statement—broad not in the sense of loose or approximate, but in that there are so many kinds of sensory and stimulus magnitudes between which are quantitative relationships susceptible of determination.

There is a relation between the frequency of a tuning fork and the pitch of its tone, between the force of an explosion and the loudness of the sound of it, between the concentration of a sugar solution and the intensity of its sweetness, between the temperature of heated copper and the quality of its color, and so on. In the vision alone, there are a great many different psychophysical relationships, each of which can be altered by various modifying factors. The relation of *true* distance and *apparent* distance, of wavelength and hue, of purity and saturation, and of energy and brightness are some of the simpler examples.

It was realized in the mid–nineteenth century that physical methods were available for precise quantitation of stimuli to the human organism. Using such precisely known stimuli, a series of workers went about studying in a systematic manner the sensation aroused in the human subject by these stimuli. By ignoring the events that transpired between stimulation of the sense organ and the production of the sensation—by treating the complex intervening mechanism as a "black box"—quantitative relationships between stimulus and response could be established.

One of the most fundamental of these is the observation by Weber in 1846[1] that the minimum detectable increment in stimulus increases as the intensity of the stimulus increases. Although Fechner[2] formulated this for several sensory modalities as $\psi = k \log \phi$ (that is, the sensation ψ is proportional to the log of the stimulus ϕ), recent workers disagree. The current formulation is that of Stevens,[3] who expresses the fundamental relationship as $\psi = k (\phi - \phi_0)^n$, sensation is proportional to the difference between the given stimulus ϕ and the threshold stimulus ϕ_0 raised to a power. The power is characteristic of the sensory modality and for the brightness of a white light is 0.33.

This is psychophysics; it represents a body of knowledge acquired over a century of study. The much more laborious problem of examining the contents of the "black box" lies in the realm of physiology. This study is still going on, but it too is beginning to offer information explaining why some of the sensations generated by the stimuli behave as they do.

Presumably, when the study of sensory physiology is complete, the psychophysical findings will flow inexorably from physiology and make a complete whole. With the present gaps in our knowledge we must consider the findings of each discipline to help explain our procedures.

The clinically practical testing methods that concern us are psychophysical testing methods in which all the stimulus variables but one are controlled and presentation simplified and shortened. This makes such tests practical in terms of time consumed, performance by the untrained patient, and precision of results no greater than is needed to indicate presence or absence of disease. However, to get a basic understanding of what underlies our clinical testing we must consider both psychophysics and physiology. This we propose to do in the following material.

THE VISUAL ACUITIES

In this section we shall learn enough about each important kind of visual acuity to get the kinds separated in our minds and to characterize each. We will then inquire more deeply into the nature of each in turn (p. 12).

Visibility acuity

When we can just see any single object that is on a background of a different character, we are making a threshold performance. The object—the "target"—may be a dot, spot, line, bar, polygon, or whatever. It may be dark or black and the ground bright or white, or vice versa. The threshold is of course the *size* of the target, if its reciprocal is to measure an "acuity." If we should keep size constant and lower intensity until the target vanished, we would be measuring an intensity threshold and a "sensitivity." The same kind of target—for example, a spot of light—obviously could be used to study both kinds of visual performance. But where *size,* not intensity or color or anything else, is the variable, the threshold size is a visibility threshold—by definition.

The stimulus "size" that we vary to find a visibility threshold may be the diameter of a dot or spot, the width *or* the length of a line, the ratio of length to width in a rectangle of constant area, and so on—just so we measure the stimulus in linear units. It is traditional, however, to convert these linear values into angular ones. The diameter of a spot on a screen subtends a certain angle at the nodal point of the observing eye and is imaged on an equal angular extent of retina. This angle is the "subtense" of the spot. The width of a "line" target has one subtense; the length of the line has another. Extensive thresholds are customarily expressed as subtenses.

The reason for this probably seems obvious. The retinal image of a 1-inch object at 2 feet has the same size as that of a 10-inch object at 20 feet; so, why not avoid having to mention the distance of the target—why not merely state its subtense, since surely it is only the size of the retinal image that matters? This is an ancient philosophy, and by and large it is a safe one. We use it in practice without exception.

However, it is worth noting that in some well-controlled experimental situations there are rare unexplained departures from visual angle constancy. These are eponymically labeled "Aubert-Forster phenomena." They do not play a role in the clinical situation.

Resolution acuity

Whenever the target consists of two or more completely separate parts between which a part of the background "shows," or when it is so shaped that the background shows through apertures in it (as with a grid) or fills a gap in it (as a break in an otherwise complete ring), one has a *resolution* situation. The observer's task is to detect the invading background within the target area or the background-filled interspace between the target's elements if these are separated, such as two parallel lines or two squares. It is not easy to teach what is meant here by "detect." Suppose, for example, that the target consists of five parallel black bars on a white ground of such length and separations that the group of bars is as wide as it is tall. The observer will be considered to be "resolving" the bars if he is able to say that the square target is not a homogenous gray patch but appears striated. He will be considered to be *proving* that he is resolving the bars if he is always correct when he says that the striations are horizontal in this target and vertical in that one. No more is asked of him—the subtense of the separation of two adjacent bars is now taken to be his resolution threshold for this particular type of target. The observer is not required to be able to count the bars or to be able to assert correctly anything about the relative widths of the bars and the interspaces between them. (Such performances would be in the category of what the French call "secondary acuities"—for which the thresholds are relatively huge.)

This may make it seem that in the measurement of resolution acuity the observer is "being let off easy." Not at all. It is only that true resolution is *defined* thus. Unfortunately, the student of physiological optics already "knows" that "visual acuity" is regularly measured with a Snellen chart, where the observer is expected to say that an E is an E—not merely that it is a nonhomogenous-looking rectangle. One needs, here and now, to try to understand that a Snellen chart does not measure a pure visual-resolution function. In the discrimination of an A from a V, resolution is less involved than the perception of the overall shapes of the letters: the testee knows that only one capital letter of the Roman alphabet can ever look like an upright triangle and that only one other letter can ever look like a triangle standing on one corner.

The simplest possible resolution target would be a pair of dots—either bright dots on a dark ground or black dots on a white ground—that one would bring closer together to find the threshold separation. The next most complex target would be a pair of fine parallel lines; next would come a pair of bars, or several lines, or several bars. The most valuable types of targets are those that afford what is called "double control." This means that the observer must not only assert that he has become aware of the "critical element" of the target but must *prove* to the experimenter that he really *is* resolving, by stating correctly *where* in the target the critical element lies or how it is oriented. For example, a square or circular patch of parallel lines offers double control, for instead of taking the observer's word for it that he is resolving the lines, one asks him to say whether the lines run horizontally, vertically, slantwise, and so on. There is some danger here. It is not unheard of for a testee to give the appearance of having low acuity, when careful questioning will elicit the information that: "But the lines ain't runnin' no place, Doc—they're just standing still."

Depending upon whether the situation is a clinical one or a "laboratory" one, double control may be invoked to keep the testee from deliberately deceiving the experimenter as to how good or how poor his resolution acuity is, or it may be used to help the testee to avoid deceiving himself. It is all too easy for even the most conscientious observer to think he is seeing something when actually he is not, and "under threshold conditions" the possibility of honest self-deception is increased to a maximum. At the same time it will usually be found, with double-control targets, that if the observer is urged to guess and is willing to do it, his performance is "better than chance." When this is the case, it is always difficult to decide what to call true threshold performance. The criterion may become just as arbitrary as it is with intensive thresholds where "50% seeing" or "60% seeing" (or almost any percentage) may be decided upon. If *pure* guesswork, with his eyes closed, would enable the observer to call correctly half of the targets in a certain line on a chart, one may decide to make the "end-point" 75%—that is, to require the observer to report three-fourths of the targets on a line correctly before calling that line of the chart his threshold line.

Among physiological optics researchers, one particular resolution target is decidedly favored over all others. This is the "Landolt ring" or "Landolt broken circle," with which double control is readily secured by presenting the ring at different times (or at different places on a chart) with the "break" oriented in any one of four, or six, or eight positions. The proportions of the genuine Landolt ring are rigidly prescribed, as seen in Fig. 1-1. Where the "stroke" of the ring (meaning the curved black line of which it is composed) is 1 unit in width and the "break" or gap is also 1 unit wide, the outside diameter of the ring is 5 units (Fig. 1-1).

The only fault of the Landolt ring is that it is not "immune to astigmatism." This means that for any observer who has even a very slight astigmatism uncorrected (and who does not?), the resolution of the gap will be favored when the gap is in particular positions in the ring, so that the observer's score will be better than it "should" be. With enough test samples at different axes, this effect can be negated.

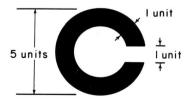

Fig. 1-1. The Landolt C and its rigidly prescribed dimensions. (Courtesy Division of Photography, Department of Medical Illustrations, J. Hillis Miller Health Center, University of Florida, Gainesville, Fla.)

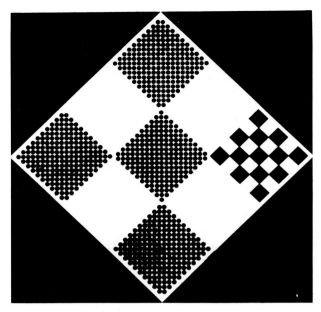

Fig. 1-2. A typical resolution challenge. (Courtesy Division of Photography, Department of Medical Illustrations, J. Hillis Miller Health Center, University of Florida, Gainesville, Fla.)

Although double control targets such as the Landolt ring require the subject to specify a direction relative to the perceived circle, it must not be thought that this test involves space perception.

The best example of the nonspatial character of resolution is the "checkerboard" target incorporated in the Bausch and Lomb Orthorater. Here each target consists of a group of four squares, one of which is different from the others. The "different" square is a black-and-white checkerboard that may contain many small squares or fewer larger ones. The other three squares are "confusion areas" —they are made to appear a smooth gray from a distance even much less than that at which the checkerboard area appears nonhomogenous (Fig. 1-2). When the subtense of the target is so small that the checkerboard appears smoothly gray, it and the confusion areas are (or are supposed to be) the same *shade* of gray. "Threshold" subtense is that at which the observer can just say which of the four squares looks somewhat different from the other three. He is then—by definition— resolving the little square elements of the checkerboard. But if he has not seen such a target under much greater subtense he will not have the slightest inkling that the "different" area is a checkerboard, let alone be able to count its elements or even to say that they are rows of squares and not rows of round spots or hexagons or what-have-you. Only if he could tell these things about the target could he be said to be perceiving its spatial organization—that is, *localizing,* in subjective visual space, each corner and side of each square in the checkerboard.

Spatial acuities

Shape (and orientation). When one *can* tell—can *barely* tell—the shape of a target (whether it is a circle, a triangle, a square, or other) one *is* making a spatial performance of a very simple kind, and the minimal subtense found to be required measures a "shape-detection acuity." If polygons with different numbers of sides (but with equal areas or fitting into a constant-sized circle) are intermingled on a chart and the subtense at which a triangle can just be "told from" a circle and that at which a square (or other) can just be told from a circle are determined, then one is measuring the thresholds of shape discrimination. More than one *kind* of threshold is involved here; the subtense at which the observer is sure that a polygon is not a circle is very different from the subtense at which he is sure that the polygon is a pentagon and not a hexagon.

Very little has ever actually been done in the way of studies of shape acuities, and still less has been done with the problems of orientation acuity. The two may seem to be one and the same performance—for, obviously, if I can barely tell that a polygon target is a triangle and not something else, I can also say (at that very same subtense) whether the triangle is apex up or apex down. But consider such a matter as the orientation of a single line, which may objectively be perfectly vertical, or a bit tilted—with the observer's task being to detect a minimal tilt. Or consider a target consisting of a pair of parallel or *almost* parallel lines, where the observer is required to decide whether they are parallel or not. Here the perception of absolute and relative orientations is involved, and there would be thresolds and their reciprocals would stand for "acuities"; but this whole field is neglected although it is certainly not unimportant. Consider how many amateur bricklayers confidently attempt to dispense with such props as stretched strings and plumblines!

Vernier acuity. Two parallel lines may be used to measure "the resolving power of the eye." The same two lines, laid end to end, can afford a measure of "the aligning power of the eye," otherwise known as *vernier acuity*, since it is the visual capacity we use when reading a vernier or nonius scale on an instrument. If one line is kept stationary and the other is made movable from side to side, a setting can be made from a just-noticeable displacement; or a series of settings for apparently perfect alignment can be made and the "sigma" of the errors calculated and taken to be the just-nonnoticeable displacement. When the displacement is expressed as an angle at the observing eye, it is a vernier threshold, and its reciprocal expresses vernier acuity (Fig. 1-3).

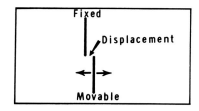

Fig. 1-3. Vernier acuity measurement with a movable line.

The simple fact that one can measure both resolution acuity and vernier acuity with two lines may make it seem that the two kinds of performance are closely related. They are often confused, but they are less related than it might appear.

It has been noted in the past that the "minimum separable" (that is, the resolution threshold) is ordinarily about 1 minute of arc. This has been correlated with the calculated diameter of the human retinal cone. Then vernier acuity, where the threshold is in the neighborhood of 4 seconds of arc, must appear paradoxical at first glance. Such resolution would seem to require stimulation of a fraction of a photoreceptor.

We are helped in our understanding of this paradox by recent work in electrophysiology. The pertinent studies on experimental animals involve the insertion of an electrode near a single cell in the retinal ganglion cell layer, in the lateral geniculate body, and in the visual cortex. By presenting various targets to the eye the shape, size, and organization of the "receptor field" corresponding to the single cell can be explored.

As outlined by Hubel,[4] the retinal ganglion cell in the cat is fed by hundreds of receptors, but the response pattern of the cell is determined by the central receptors in the field. Stimulation of the center of the field of the "on-center" type cell causes firing. The "off-center" type cell is inhibited by light to the center of its field; in each case light falling outside the center of the field alters the on or off response given by the field center. This is obviously a contrast-sharpening mechanism. At the lateral geniculate body this effect is pyramided. On-center and off-center organization are preserved. One particular optic nerve fiber (that is, one ganglion cell) triggers a single lateral geniculate cell, but diffuse illumination of the surrounding field causes very little response. Thus the contrast is sharpened still farther.

Finally, in the striate cortex the receptive field of any given cell has a *linear* distribution rather than radial one. There are narrow excitatory linear fields surrounded by inhibitory fields, or inhibitory fields surrounded by excitatory fields, or bipartite fields where excitation and inhibition meet at a linear boundary. The inclination of the line defining the field of a given cortical cell is constant, of course. However, cells exist with lines at all inclinations and none appear to be favored more than others.

It is the combination of contrast sharpening and linear organization that explains the high sensitivity of vernier acuity. All images falling on the retina are blurred by diffraction and the optical aberrations of the eye. This blurring is combated by the image-sharpening mechanisms just described. This much works as effectively for resolution as for vernier acuity. But beyond this, if you wanted to pick the most sensitive resolution task on the basis of cortical organization, you would pick precisely the vernier problem. Because of the linear organization of cortical receptor fields, the alignment problem should be the most sensitive test of resolution. One day a clairvoyant psychophysicist might have postulated this neural organization on the basis of the long-known psychophysical findings. The invasion of the interior of the "black box" by physiologists is the more direct approach.

Motion. The visual perception of an object *as being in motion* is really a perception of a continuously changing direction. Obviously, if the observer is stationary and his eyeball is also stationary, an object moving vertically or laterally across his visual field lies in one after another of a series of receptor fields. These fields are finite in number, as the existence of a *finite* vernier threshold shows. By that same token it might be expected that the angular threshold of motion would agree closely with the vernier threshold. With similar targets and under the proper conditions, it does.

The most important of these conditions is the angular velocity at which the target moves across the visual field. For this velocity itself there are *two* "threshold" values and still a third critical value between the lower and upper threshold. If an object moves at less than a certain *lower threshold* speed across the field (expressed in minutes of arc per second of time), it cannot be seen to move. In the case of such an object as the hour hand of a clock, one may *know* that it is in motion, and one's evidence for this may be purely visual—*seeing* from time to time that the hand is in new positions. This is not, however, the visual perception of motion, for this means perceiving the *motion,* the *moving.* It is the direct detection of a changing of position (direction) that constitutes "visual movements."

At the other end of the scale, if the speed of an object is increased indefinitely, a point is reached when the object cannot be seen clearly enough to be identifiable without foreknowledge of what it is. However, an observer will still see that something has crossed his field and will know whether it went from left to right or in some other path. Since *an* object (unknown) is being seen to be in motion, visual movement is still being experienced. But when the speed is such that the object can cross the field of view before the impression of it in its position of first appearance has had time to fade, the *upper threshold* velocity has been attained. The observer no longer sees an object, let alone an object "going thataway." If he even still knows that "something went by," it will always be found that his knowledge is based upon nonvisual information.

For a given sort of object or target, there is always an angular velocity lying between the lower and upper limits at which the visual movement is seen best. It may seem that there would be no very critical value for "best" seeing. But there is one, if by "best" we mean the situation where the just-visible extent of movement is as low as it can be made. This is to say, there is an *optimal* velocity for the target at which one will find the lowest value for the angular threshold of motion. Indeed, the angular threshold has to be defined and measured under optimal velocity conditions, else the value found means nothing.

If a target *is* moving at optimal *velocity* and is exposed for only the length of time it requires to travel through the threshold *angle,* that length of time can be considered to be a *durational* threshold of visual motion. It is the minimum time the object must be in motion in order to be capable of being seen in motion. This "third" threshold is not at all independent of the other two. There are reciprocal relationships that can be defined accurately.

To an extent perhaps greater than with any other kind of visual acuity, motion acuity is influenced by the character of the target. Its size has greater effect, and so does its intensitive contrast with the background. An ordinary bullet is apparently too small to be seen in motion at its high velocity—but a tracer bullet, no larger, is easily visible because it is so bright. A shell from a 3-inch field artillery piece cannot be seen to travel. One from a 16-inch naval rifle on a battleship, although it travels faster, can be seen in transit because it is so large.

The presence of stationary landmarks cuts all motion thresholds practically in half. Movement is much more readily detected when it is movement of an object *relative* to another (motionless) object and *near* the other object. "Relativity" is important to the perception of motion in another way also: the perception of relative motion is fraught with "illusions" as regards *which* of the objects is the one in motion and which is the one standing still. The "railroad illusion" is the most familiar illustration of this, but laboratory demonstrations in a dark-room can be even more impressive. Here where only one of two lights is really moving, the motion is very likely to be attributed to the *other* light if the latter is much the smaller, or the brighter, of the two.

Stereoacuity. Stereoscopic visual acuity—the ability of a subject to determine distance differences using stereoscopic cues—is measured in the office in a very approximate manner. For a treatment of the practical aspects of depth perception including stereopsis, see Chapter 7.

BASES OF THE ACUITIES
Visibility

With bright-on-dark targets. The simplest imaginable visibility situation would offer an illuminated patch in a field of darkness. With intensity held constant, a threshold subtense could be found for the patch. Suppose its size is then held constant at threshold and the intensity is reduced a little. The spot will disappear. Raising the intensity will cause it to reappear. If now the spot is made smaller than threshold size, it vanishes; however, a further rise in intensity will restore it to visibility.

In this situation, it is obvious that when a threshold size is determined for a spot, this is tantamount to determining the *absolute intensity threshold* for a spot of that size. Indeed, it will be found that there is no true threshold *size* for the spot; for, whenever a shrinking spot becomes invisible, it can be made to reappear merely by raising its intensity. No matter how small the retinal image of the spot may be, it can always affect some receptors if it contains enough energy.

At this point, a fundamental fact must be made abundantly clear. We can talk all we want about neat geometrical retinal image points, conjugate optically to each point in the object of regard—but such a situation is only a convenient way to teach geometrical optics and is only roughly related to *actual* retinal images. To know what the true image of every point in space is really like on our retinas, we must understand the physical phenomenon of diffraction.

Diffraction. Diffraction is the ability of light to apparently "bend around corners" or appear in areas of an image or shadow where you don't expect to see it on strictly geometrical optics reasoning (Fig. 1-4).

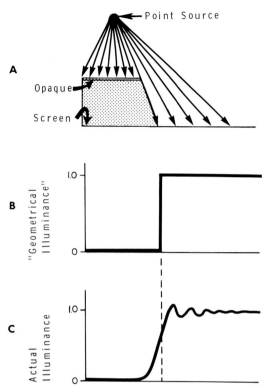

Fig. 1-4. Diagram illustrating diffraction by a sharp edge. **A,** A point source casts a geometrically sharp shadow on a screen; **B,** the *theoretical* illuminance of that shadow; **C,** the *actual* illuminance of the shadow (diffraction pattern).

The effect of diffraction is negligible if you consider *large* openings and large distances relative to the minute wavelength of light. Thus, if you are considering the *macroscopic* effects of light—that is, the light focusing effects of a lens system, the optical components of the eye, or object-image relationships—these can be quite adequately described in terms of strict geometrical optics and the *refraction* of light, based on Snell's law. However, when one considers the "microscopic" aspects of light (such as the finer details of retinal image illumination), account must be taken of *diffraction*. Even when light passes through as large an opening as the pupil of the eye, the retinal image is, in reality, the diffracted image of that source—light has to "squeeze" through the pupil before it falls on the retina.

The diffraction image of even a tiny source of light has the appearance of a central "hot spot" surrounded by a series of bright, regularly spaced rings, each decreasing in intensity (Fig. 1-5). If the source is not a point but an extended object, there is a diffraction image corresponding to *every* point making up the object.

Intensity of diffraction pattern

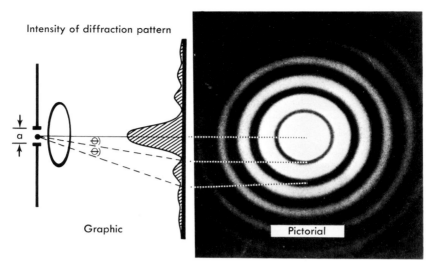

Graphic

Pictorial

Fig. 1-5. The diffraction pattern with a circular opening. (Courtesy Division of Photography, Department of Medical Illustrations, J. Hillis Miller Health Center, University of Florida, Gainesville, Fla.)

Diffraction can occur only when a light beam passes by an opaque object. Thus, we are constantly aware of its effects in any optical instrument, where light is almost always impeded by apertures. The diffraction pattern produced by them will determine the limiting sharpness of the image. With circular apertures, such as the pupils, the angular separation θ (in radians) between the center of the "bright spot" and the first *dark* ring is equal to the angular separation of each of the succeeding *dark* rings (Fig. 1-5).

$$\theta = 1.22 \frac{\lambda}{a}$$

Where θ = angular separation (in radians) at the
center of the aperture
λ = the wavelength of light
a = diameter of the aperture

The diffraction pattern is obviously larger with smaller pupil diameters and has visual significance with pupils less than about 2.5 mm. (Visual acuity is actually decreased somewhat when one looks through a 1-mm pinhole because of the diffraction effect caused by the pinhole; see p. 25.) Even when one deals with large openings or slits, if the edge of the light pattern in the image (in shadow) is closely examined, the effect of diffraction can be noticed (Fig. 1-4).

Thus the diffraction image of even a theoretical point source of light has *finite* size and is spread out over many receptors. This can be shown as follows:

The angular size in radians of the total "hot spot" of the diffraction image on the retina of a distant point source of light (with the pupil at 3.0 mm and light of $\lambda 555$ nm) is

$$\theta = 2 \ (1.22) \times \frac{\lambda}{a}$$

$$\theta = 2 \times \frac{1.22 \ (555 \times 10^{-6} \ m)}{3.0}$$

$$\theta = 450 \times 10^{-6} \ \text{radians} = 1.62 \ \text{minutes of arc}$$

This corresponds to an overall length on the retina of

$$17 \times 450 \times 10^{-6} \ mm = 0.0077 \ mm$$

$$= 7.7 \ \mu$$

Since the known diameter of the outer segment of a macular cone is about 1.1μ, the true retinal image of any "point" source is actually spread out and could stimulate about *seven* foveal cones (and this calculation considers only the size of the *central* "hot spot" of the diffraction image!).

Raising the intensity of the point source will *not* enlarge the overall image, but the energy in a receptor-sized area at the center of the "hot spot" of the diffraction image need only to be above a certain minimum threshold to effectively stimulate at *least* one receptor (see Fig. 1-8); in the fovea, one receptor can be responsible for a sensation.

Precisely the same considerations pertain to the visibility of a bright line on a dark field. There is no threshold width for such a line if intensity is not limited. Visibility acuity becomes "infinite." At least, it is physically impossible to make a bright line (in the form of a slit between pieces of metal) capable of being narrowed far enough (without "breaking up") to find a threshold width when the slit is placed between the eye and an intense source. Niven and Brown[5] plotted log "threshold" width against log intensity and obtained a straight line.

The situation is not much different when the background of a bright spot or line is not totally dark but contains some illumination. What now limits the just-visible size of the target is the *differential intensity threshold*. As the retinal image of the target shrinks, the retinal illuminance provided by the extensive field does not change, but the increment of illuminance provided by the target falls. When it is no more than a $\triangle I$ value above the field illuminance, the threshold width of the target has been reached. The target can, however, be made still narrower and still be seen if its intensity is raised enough to restore a $\triangle I$ difference between the most intense and least intense portions of the whole retinal image of target and field.

Bright-on-dark and bright-on-less-bright "visibility" configuration of targets and grounds thus merely test the absolute and differential intensity functions of the observer in circumstances such that spatial dimensions are "limiting." They measure no visual functions that in themselves are essentially "spatial." This is further emphasized when *time* is allowed to become a variable, along with intensity and retinal area stimulated. Suppose we consider the situation where area has been made very small, intensity (either absolute or incremental) has been made very low, and time (duration of stimulation) has been made very brief. Suppose now that the observer is seeing 50% of all such stimuli. "A" threshold has been found, but, a threshold value of *what?* Area? No, for we can increase either intensity or time, *reduce* area, and still see 50% of the flashes.

Intensity? No, for we can increase area or time, *decrease* intensity, and still see. Time? Again, we can see despite a further reduction of time, provided we increase either area or intensity.

Intensity, area, and time are thus in a way "interchangeable" within certain limits and *jointly* determine threshold performance. This must be because there is some one quantity that all three variables are causing to vary, and the true threshold is a threshold value of this quantity. The quantity in question must be the *total luminous* flux being received by the retina. This would be the *time* × the time-rate of flow of light (= the flux) per unit area (= the illuminance, the *intensity*) × the area. For a threshold sensory effect, what is necessary is a critical value of the triple product of intensity, area, and time.

This is hardly astounding in view of the known neural connections in retina and geniculate body described previously. However, it must be understood that the final psychophysical result is conditioned on summations and differentiations at at least five different levels (outer nuclear, ganglion cell, lateral geniculate, calcarine cortex, visual association areas). The psychophysical end result is an overall final product. It does not allow specific conclusions about the intervening machinery. For time to be able to replace intensity and/or area means that the effects, within a receptor, of absorbing repeated doses of quanta are the same as if the same total number of quanta had been absorbed as one dose, provided all the doses arrive within a period so brief that the intrareceptoral effect of the first dose (inadequate, in itself, to cause a sensation) has not begun to wear off. There is, then, *temporal* summation as well as *areal* summation.

These kinds of summation are separately expressed in two laws, the relationship between which could not be seen until relatively recently: the Bunsen-Roscoe law and Ricco's law. The Bunsen-Roscoe law states that for a constant amount of photochemical effect, it is only necessary for the product of intensity × time to be a constant. It is because the latent image in a photographic emulsion obeys this law that "time exposures" are possible with a camera. Time can substitute indefinitely for intensity. In vision, however, the retina obeys the law so long as the time does not exceed 0.02 second. For durations less than this, the "intensity threshold" depends upon the stimulation time and the real threshold is some constant product of intensity × time. This is true not only in rod vision but also for cone-threshold performance within the fovea. A television engineer would say that 0.02 second represents the maximum "storage time" possible for the visual "pickup device."

Ricco formulated *his* law in 1877. It holds good within a foveocentral area of about 50 minutes subtense and remains approximately true within an area as large as 2.5 degrees. It states that for a given area, the threshold intensity will be such that intensity × area is a constant. The breakdown of Ricco's law outside the fovea led Haig (1948) to suspect that if the threshold situation were put on a basis not of raw retinal area involved but of the totalized cross-sectional areas of the *receptors* in that area, the law might not break down. To be able to make comparisons between peripheral and foveal areas, Haig restricted his consideration to cone threshold conditions. He reasoned that if Ricco's law holds for the pure cone spot in the fovea 50 minutes in diameter, then it should hold in the periphery for an area large enough to contain so many cones that these—if they were contiguous—would just fill up a 50-minute spot. If the area of a patch of retina is called *a* and the total cross-sectional area of the cones in it is called *s*, then s/a is the fraction of *a* comprised by cones. At the center of the fovea, of course s/a = 1. What Haig did was to stimulate various places in the periphery where comparable histological situations were on record. He found that within an area *a* the required intensity (I) is always such that I × s/a = k, a constant. The value of *a* could of course be much larger, in the periphery, than the 50-minute spot within which Ricco's law holds strictly true in the fovea. Haig's apparatus allowed him to make his determinations only as far as 18 degrees into the periphery, but he saw no reason to think that his modification of Ricco's law would not hold anywhere on the retina.

"Haig's law"—if we wish to call it that—supersedes Ricco's law. Thus, we can, if we like, speak of a "Bunsen-Roscoe-Haig law" subsuming both areal and temporal summations. For, clearly, for constant threshold visibility in small area, with brief exposures, the equation I × t × s/a = K will be found to apply. This equation, or "law," merely says that the true threshold is a particular amount of total flux intercepted by the visual cells. This is really only "to be expected."

With black-on-white targets. When a visibility target is darker than the ground, the intensity discrimination function (ΔI/I versus log I) still governs the performance, just as in the case of a bright-on-a-less-bright target ground situation. Superficially, there is an enormous difference between the two situations, for with a dark-on-a-less-dark, or black-on-white, configuration there is a finite threshold width of spot or line that can be seen, no matter how intensely the field is illuminated. It may seem paradoxical to assert that "ΔI/I" (contrast) is involved in the seeing of a *black* line on a *white* ground, for the contrast between the two is already "maximal."

The objective contrast between a black spot or line and its white background is indeed high and is *not* changed by making the line narrower and narrower, indefinitely. But, for visibility, what counts is not the contrast of the *real* object but the contrast in the patient's retinal image between the line part and the field part. The diffraction image of the line-and-ground configuration is actually a pattern of retinal illuminances (Fig. 1-6), with illuminance not zero anywhere (corresponding to "black") unless the target line is many times threshold width. Each edge or "side" of the target line is responsible (via diffraction) for a falling-off of retinal illuminance along a certain course. The summation of these distributions gives the real distribution of light in the retinal image in a "section" passing from the clear field image through the line image to the field on the other side of the line. The line image is actually a mere "dip" in the illuminance from the field illuminance, (I_f) to some lower value (I_d). Obviously, I_d could not become zero unless the target line were made very wide. As the line is made narrower, the "dip" becomes shallower: I_d approaches I_f. The contrast in the image, at any time, equals $(I_f - I_d)/I_d$. When I_d is just discriminable from I_f, we have the familiar situation in which $(I_2 - I_1)/I_1 = \Delta$I/I. This will be the situation for some particular width of line, at any given value of I_f. But increasing I_f will not

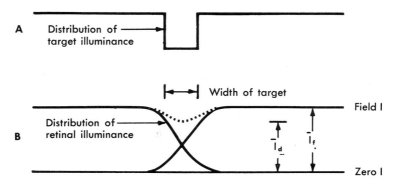

Fig. 1-6. The pattern of a black line on a white background. **A,** Geometrical *target* illuminance; **B,** actual *retinal* illuminance. (Courtesy Division of Photography, Department of Medical Illustrations, J. Hillis Miller Health Center, University of Florida, Gainesville, Fla.)

change the relationship of I_f to I_d—it will not change the contrast. If the intensity of the field (giving I_f) has been carried as high as gives the minimal value of $\Delta I/I$ (0.006), and the line is narrowed until $(I_f - I_d)/I_d$ equals this minimal value, the width of the line is now an irreducible visibility threshold. To raise I_f any higher will not make it possible to see a narrower line, for a narrower line will make $(I_f - I_d)/I_d$ a subliminal value of contrast.

This reasoning was confirmed experimentally by Hecht and Mintz in 1939. They viewed black wires stretched across a transilluminated opal glass disk and determined the size of wire that was just visible when the luminance of the disk had various values up to 30 mL. The threshold subtense of the wire turned out to be 0.44 second (arc) at their highest intensity, and as much as 10 minutes at their lowest. They calculated the corresponding distributions of illuminance across the retinal image and were easily able to show that for each I_f and each threshold subtense, $(I_f - I_d)/I_d$ always corresponded to the (same) value of $\Delta I/I$. The visibility of the black line is thus a mere special case of intensity discrimination. It is just one expression of the observer's contrast sensitivity, which is of course his personal maximal value of $\Delta I/I$.

The visibility of a black "dot"—a circular black spot—on a white ground has exactly the same basis. Here, however, the threshold subtense of the spot seems very large as compared with the threshold substense of line. Round-spot visibility has been studied off and on for a century, but the results of all investigations are in excellent agreement: 30 seconds, 32 seconds, 34 seconds and so on. In the light of our knowledge of the special organization of the calcarine cortex, this is a highly logical finding.

Two factors are, however, known for sure to be capable of reducing the threshold width of a spot, even after the intensity of the field has been raised to optimum. *Irregularity* helps, and so (within limits) does *motion*. For a black *square* on a 1,000-mL field, the threshold subtense is claimed to be only 9 seconds, compared with 30 seconds or more for a black circle. The "corners" of the target image subject the receptors to particularly rapid *changes* in stimulation owing to the fine involuntary vibrations of the eye during "fixation." This is as important, for discrimination, as the static difference between I_f and I_d in a retinal image imagined to be motionless. For related reasons, *some* movement (not too far or too fast) of a visibility target will lower the size threshold. The image continuously encounters fresh receptors and leaves them behind before they have had time to adapt to it.*

An important and interesting consideration in connection with visibility is the manner in which the appearance of a visibility target changes as its subtense is progressively reduced to and finally below threshold value. Suppose the target is a black line on a white ground. When the line is wide, it *appears* black and its width can be estimated. As the subtense is reduced, the line is *seen* to become thinner, but during this process it will eventually begin to lose "contrast" and to become "gray." As the line becomes visibly thinner, the gray becomes visibly lighter or paler. The perceptual thinning of the line slows up and comes to a halt, although the objective narrowing of the target line is steadily continuing.

At this point, the line looks as narrow as it ever will, although the width of the objective line is still above threshold. The line row has its "minimal apparent width." As the target is further reduced in subtense, the only further change of the perceived line is a further loss of contrast with the ground. At threshold, the line is of such a pale gray that it is just barely not white; the line finally vanishes, not by narrowing to zero width but by bleaching to zero contrast.

This situation was studied quantitatively by the photographic opticist, Lapicque, in 1938. He devised a target comprised of two lines or bars of equal length but with one twice as wide as the other and having half the contrast of the narrower line. When this entire target is reduced in subtense, a point is reached where both lines have the *same* apparent width; this is *minimal* for each line. From this subtense on down to threshold subtense, the halves of the target remain constant in apparent width and are always alike in grayness, so that the observer cannot tell which end of the target is rightmost (Fig. 1-7).

Lapicque calculated the curves of the distribution of retinal illuminance across the retinal images of the two lines. He was able to show that at minimal apparent width the two curves were identical, since the difference in objective contrast of the lines was exactly compensated by their difference in objective width. This explained why the two lines were seen as *equal* in width.

With spots or "points" of light, the phenomenon of minimal apparent width accounts for the appearances of, for example, stars. The *actual* diameters of various stars vary greatly but are utterly unrelated to the *apparent* sizes of the stars, which, as we have seen, are dependent on the retinal image diffraction patterns. The earliest astronomers did not know this and classified stars as to their "mag-

---

*An image that stands perfectly still on the retina may "fade" because of adaptation. It will soon reappear, seemingly spontaneously, but probably always because a blink or some other act has caused a slight eye movement. If one spot in a small constellation of well-spaced black spots is fixated, it will be noted that each other spot disappears temporarily from time to time ("Troxler's phenomenon").[21] The dramatic work with the stabilized retinal image done by Ditchburn in England and Riggs in the United States is the best demonstration of this phenomenon.

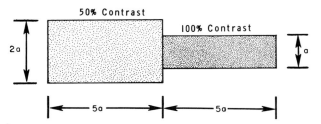

Fig. 1-7. When this target is reduced in subtense, a size will be reached when both the right and left sections will appear to have the same width. (Courtesy Division of Photography, Department of Medical Illustrations, J. Hillis Miller Health Center, University of Florida, Gainesville, Fla.)

nitudes"—which were intended to be taken literally to *mean* sizes. The telescope, however, eventually showed that "magnitude" went with *intensity* and not with subtense. The term has remained in use to this day as an *intensity* label.

A star of the lowest visible magnitude has minimal apparent width. It effectively stimulates only one foveal cone—one cone *at a time*, that is, for visual fixation is not rock steady! A star of any high magnitude is merely one so intense that its retinal image provides supraliminal illuminance over an area containing *several* cones. With a constant size of pupil, the diffraction images of two different "point sources" of different candlepower are *not* different in *diameter*, but the curves of the distribution of illuminance in them are different in heights (Fig. 1-8).

When a point source is *very* intense, its apparent size becomes even larger than that of a less-intense source that stimulates, supraliminally, the same number of receptors. There are two factors in the reason for this. Light *scattered* within the retinal tissue can activate receptors outside the confines of the actual image. This is "irradiation" of the same, purely physical, sort that can occur in the emulsion on a photographic film. Then there is a *neural* "irradiation" that is actually much more important: ganglion cells outside of an intense image are brought into action by horizontal and/or amacrine cells within the image, so that the effect upon apparent size is exactly as if the receptors immediately above those ganglion cells were being stimulated by light. The total irradiation has its greatest visual importance in connection with the resolution of bright target elements on a dark ground, as we shall shortly see.

Resolution

With bright-on-dark targets. The *resolvability* of a pair of bright squares, bars, or lines on a dark ground is identical—so far as one can tell—with the basis of the *visibility* of a dark line on a bright ground. When the elements of the target are pushed together until the observer can just see a shadowy line of demarcation between them, this line represents a threshold extent of contrast in the retinal image, between the interspace part and the element parts of the image. The performance is a special case of intensity discrimination.

The effect of the intensity of the target elements upon their threshold sep-

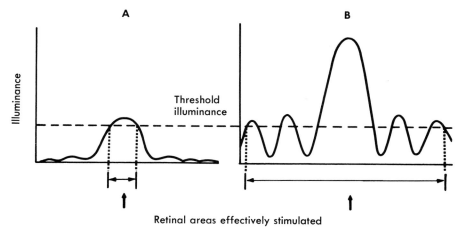

Fig. 1-8. The retinal diffraction image of a "point" source. **A,** Above threshold intensity, but barely so; **B,** of higher intensity. It appears "larger," though the "point" source is the same size in both cases. (Courtesy Division of Photography, Department of Medical Illustrations, J. Hillis Miller Health Center, University of Florida, Gainesville, Fla.)

aration is somewhat unexpected. One expects to see better and better as illumination is elevated. But with bright dots or squares, resolvability *deteriorates* as intensity is raised, and with large bright bars the performance improves for a time and then deteriorates, so that there is an optimum intensity that gives a minimum threshold separation.

The cause of a *decrease* in resolvability with an increase in intensity is quite obvious; it is irradiation. Each of the target elements appears to expand as its intensity is raised, so that the dark retinal interspace is filled in with "light" and is obliterated. If, however, one starts at a sufficiently low intensity, it is found that as intensity is raised, large areas *shrink* for a time before they begin to expand. The intensity at the turning point is the optimal one for resolution. Irradiation can thus be said to be sometimes *negative* at low intensities. This was discovered long ago by Volkmann; its explanation lies in the contrast-enhanced interaction of retinal elements described before.

Bright-on-dark resolution acuity is never very "good." Resolution charts and targets that are identical, except for being related to each other like a photographic positive to its negative, are consequently *not* interchangeable. The observer's performance will be poorer, other things being equal, with the chart presenting bright-on-dark situations. The average threshold separation of two black dots on a bright ground is usually taken to be 1 minute of arc. The threshold for bright dots on a dark field (for example, stars in the night sky) is said to be about 3 minutes for the average observer. (This corresponds to a Snellen acuity of about 20/60.)

With black-on-white targets. It cannot be too strongly emphasized that for black elements on a bright ground the whole nature of the performance (hence, its physiological basis) profoundly depends upon the characters of element con-

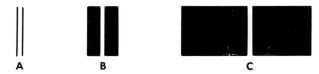

Fig. 1-9. Three resolution targets. (Courtesy Division of Photography, Department of Medical Illustrations, J. Hillis Miller Health Center, University of Florida, Gainesville, Fla.)

stellations employed. What is a clear-cut resolution performance in one situation may be changed by imperceptible degrees into a performance that is not resolution at all, merely by making a "simple, quantitative" change in the shape of the target. Consider Fig. 1-9: the lines at *A*, the bars at *B*, and the blocks at *C* all have the same height and the same separation. But the interspace is much more easily resolved in *B* than in *A* and far more easily in *C* than even in *B*. In *C* the observer's actual problem is the *visibility* of a bright line on a dark ground—for which, as we have said, there is *no* threshold width. Where along the road from *A* to *C* has the stiuation changed from a resolution situation to a visibility situation? No one would like to have to say. But this demonstration, that resolution intergrades with other kinds of performance having vastly different thresholds, goes to show that whenever an individual's "visual acuity" is stated, the target used to measure it should be mentioned in the same breath.

The "optical resolving power" of the eye,* as calculated with the criterion employed in the past, was about 1 minute (64 seconds). Everything fitted nicely to prove that there had to be an unstimulated cone between two stimulated ones if two points were to be resolved. We are still feeling the effects of this doctrine—for are we not still using the Snellen and Landolt characters, whose "critical details" were designed to subtend 1 minute at 6 meters?

It is only necessary to substitute real diffraction retinal images for imaginary geometrical-optical ones to see at once that the size of a foveal cone cannot possibly determine the resolution threshold as a value equal to itself. It is only necessary for the receptor(s) "in the middle" to receive perceptibly *less,* or *more,* stimulation than the adjacent ones for resolution to occur. It was Hoffman and (independently) Hartridge[6] who first perceived this and set the matter forth in the early 1920's. The theory, or viewpoint, that resolution is only a special case of intensity discrimination or contrast sensitivity, with the intensities discriminated being illuminances in different parts of the retinal image, dates from this work. The *best* theory of black-on-white resolutions and its relations to intensity is still this contrast sensitivity theory of Hartridge, which considers resolution to be retinal image intensity discrimination (modern modifications by

---

*The resolving power of an optical instrument has no physiological implication and in fact has no meaning or value whatever, save as a basis for comparing the instrument with another instrument of the same sort. The determination of resolving power always involved an *assumed* value for visual contrast sensitivity, which is never realistic. The "Raleigh criterion," by which resolving power was calculated from the 1880's until just lately, assumed $\Delta I/I \times 100 = 13\%$ (whereas it is 1% or less). On this basis, an opticist can "prove" that the human eye's resolution threshold could not possibly be less than 42 seconds of arc!

Shlaer[7] and Hendley[8]). On the other hand, O'Brien[9] in 1951 has presented evidence that the previously mentioned hypothesis fails to explain completely the observed change in foveal visual acuity with general retinal illumination. The complex supraretinal organization of the visual system probably accounts for this.

Yet another modification to Hartridge's theory was that of Toraldo di Francia.[10] The spread of light in the diffraction image of two stars is the sum of that in the two individual images. At threshold separation, one detects the $\triangle I$ of the central dip between the two "humps" for a given level of retinal illuminance; the observer then barely detects *two* stars. If the two stars move closer together, their images move closer together and will yield a retinal light distribution that, although exhibiting a single hump, may differ just enough from that given by a *single* star that the subject may be able to identify the existence of *two* stars. This improved performance, which yields "threshold" measurements smaller than expected, is caused by the a priori knowledge that the possible stimulus situations were limited to two—one star or two stars. Had the observer not known this before attempting the discrimination, he would not be able to differentiate between a single, elliptical light and a double star. Thus the prior awareness of the existence of only two choices definitely increases the probability of detection of a smaller $\triangle I$ than is otherwise possible.

Recently considerable emphasis has been placed on the use of sinusoidal gratings as test objects and on the implications of the findings obtained.[11-13] A sinusoidal grating is one in which density varies as the sine of the distance along one dimension and is constant along a second dimension at right angles to the first. The virtues are, first, that despite optical aberrations and absorption in the ocular media a sinusoidal test grating will produce a true sinusoidal image on the retina. The second virtue is that the retinal image can be analyzed by well-established mathematical methods introduced by Fourier and used in optics and in control systems.

Thus the retinal image may be described in terms of the "modulation transfer function": the change in contrast as a function of the number of sinusoidal cycles per unit distance. Actual experimental measurements have been made of the "line spread function" by photometry of the ophthalmoscopic image. An equivalent function can be calculated for the sinusoidal target.

When such targets are used for psychophysical studies where the whole neural pathway is inserted into the experiment, a threshold is obtained for resolution that varies with amount of contrast (modulation) of the grating and with the number of cycles per unit of visual angle. This is expected. However, for targets above 10 minutes of arc per cycle, these targets are paradoxically less resolvable. This is not explicable on the basis of Fourier theory and is obviously a property of neural organization.

FACTORS AFFECTING RESOLUTION
Illumination and luminance

Several factors have been shown to affect resolution acuity for better or for worse. The most conspicuous one, which everyone should know about, is intensity of illumination. This operates not by changing the relative luminances of target and ground but primarily by changing the value of $\Delta I/I$. However, by raising intensity, one gets only a slight return in increased acuity. A factor of 200% has a negligible effect; so, why read under 40 ft-c when 20 ft-c costs only half as much? One is never trying to read *threshold* print anyway! Acuity increases roughly as the logarithm of the intensity. Gilbert and Hopkinson (1949) found that with Snellen charts the illuminance had to be increased from 0.1 to 1.0 ft-c to raise acuity by one line.

In your refracting lanes, then, use good, even, target illumination of between 5 and 20 ft-c. Also, assure comparability of acuity measurements from one refracting lane to another by having comparable illuminances of the charts used. Keep your Project-O-Chart bulbs fresh.

Adaptation

Lythgoe[14] thoroughly investigated the effect of the adaptation state of the eye on visual acuity measurement. More recently Brown[15] has tabulated the differences in test field luminances necessary for the subject to detect light and to resolve grating targets of various resolution challenges during the course of dark adaptation. A conclusion is that acuity is certainly influenced by the *general* illumination falling on the retina. This is so even when the effect of the increased illumination on the pupil is considered. Thus the implication is that it is important to maintain the retina of the patient being refracted in a light-adapted state, *not* in semi-dark adaptation, as is usually the case.

Target type and situation

We have already discussed and will later further elaborate the marked variation in legibility (visibility) of the various letters of a Snellen chart.

Further, unexpected things happen when a row of dots or a series of parallel lines is used as a target instead of a single pair of dots or lines. Resolution becomes poorer, and the threshold agrees closely with the center-to-center separation of foveal cones. The serially repeated retinal image must be "in registry" with the cone mosaic, and the built-in contrast-enhancing mechanism is nullified. Curiously, the number of lines "per inch" that can be resolved is independent of considerable variation in the relative widths of the lines and the interspaces. Grille targets are common on visual acuity charts but can be unsatisfactory not only because they measure the visual cells rather than the visual acuity but because they are particularly sensitive to astigmatism. This is particularly evident in that grating acuity is much higher in vertical and horizontal as against oblique target orientations. Thus acuity judgments with such targets require multiple orientation at each acuity level.

One should not lose sight of the fact that there is nothing about resolution per se that demands that it have its basis in intensity differences in the target and in the retinal image. It is perfectly possible to set up a resolution target consisting of a pair of red lines on a green ground, for example. It is possible, again, to make the lines and ground exactly equal in intensity and still "resolve" them. *This* kind of resolution has never been thoroughly studied.

Motion of the target has interesting effects because of the fact that by preventing local adaptation, motion keeps the brightnesses of target and ground from "equalizing." If the target has a simple pattern, it is resolved better when in motion than when stationary, but the opposite is true for complex targets. Related to these effects is the fact that resolution is always better in a brief glance at any target than it is in a prolonged stare.

"Glare" is usually regarded as detrimental, but a glare source well off the visual axis can actually increase visual acuity by closing the pupil farther than the light received by the eyes from the visual task would do. "Veiling glare," or light reflected specularly by the visual material into the eyes, lowers the contrasts in the retinal image and lowers visual acuity accordingly. The old rule for avoiding veiling glare in a reading situation is to lay a mirror on the reading matter. If you can see a light source in the mirror, move the lamp (or yourself) until you cannot.

Pupil

The blur circles in the retinal image, because of diffraction, become larger with a small pupil and smaller with a larger pupil. On the contrary the blur circles caused by spherical and chromatic aberration vary directly with the size of the pupil. Hence, there is an *optimal* size of pupil that gives the sharpness of the image its nearest approach to that of the fictitious, geometrical-optical "point" image. Visual acuity is consequently maximal over a certain range of pupil diameters. Theoretically, this range is from 3 to 6 mm. The "physiological" size of the pupil—its usual size under photopic conditions—is about 4 mm.

In the earliest work on the effect of pupil size upon visual acuity, Hummelsheim (1898) varied intensity from 0.1 to 18 mL. The normal pupil varied in diameter from 4.0 to 7.25 mm. Under nicotine, the pupils of Hummelsheim's subjects varied from 1.5 to 2.75 mm and the visual acuities were higher than with normal pupils. Under mydriatics, the pupils were 8.75 mm in diameter and visual acuities were lower than with undrugged pupils. Lister (the inventor of antiseptic surgery) used artificial pupils and found acuity to be almost constant for diameters from 2.54 to 6.1 mm, but slightly superior for a diameter of 4.0 mm. Cobb[16] found acuity to be highest with 3.0- to 4.0-mm pupils but constant from 2.0 to 5.0 mm when retinal illuminance was made constant. Many optical instruments provide an artificial pupil (the "exit pupil") 2.0 mm in diameter. It should be closer to 3.0 mm.

When a *refractive* error exists, decreasing the pupil size will decrease the size of the blur circles on the retina and will almost always increase the visual acuity performance if the target is bright enough. But this improvement will only be to the level attainable by an emmetropic eye with the comparably sized pupil because of the diffraction effect. Thus, if you use a 0.75-mm pinhole to check for refractive anomaly (with 100 ft-c chart illumination), do not expect more than a maximum Snellen acuity of about 20/40.

Refractive state

Since, clinically, acuity and refractive corrections go hand in glove, the specific influence of refractive error on visual acuity has been a frequent problem for researchers in physiological optics: the least perceptible differences in dioptric power that can be discriminated, the effect of optical blurring on the eye's contrast thresholds and perimetric thresholds, and countless others have been extensively investigated but need not be gone into here.

Even small, uncorrected spherical refractive errors have a considerable effect on visual acuity measurements, but the effect is lessened at high intensities. Astigmatism affects acuity, but the effect depends upon the orientation of the target. It should be obvious, then, that before you should attempt to measure a visual acuity for an industrial commission report, for example, you must have the patient fully corrected with an *optimal* corrective lens. Too often a glib acuity is stated when it is recorded only with the patient's *current* lenses with no further refinement.

Wavelength of stimuli

Quite apart from the incidental fact that they happen to afford color sensations, two different monochromatic or polychromatic illuminations may give different visual acuities. The effect is, largely, purely optical—by way of chromatic aberration—and would be the same for a dichromat or for an atypical achromat as for a person with normal color vision.

In commonplace vision with white illumination, one is not aware of any "color fringes" on objects. They are demonstrable only by special means, such as by covering half of the pupil. But the factors that suppress their *colors* in ordinary vision do not suppress their *widths* and the effect thereof upon the blurredness of the retinal image. It is often said—but is not true—that since we do not see the fringes, chromatic aberration has a negligible deteriorative effect upon the sharpness of the retinal image and upon visual acuity. In white light, the foci of the ends of the spectrum are separated on the optic axis of the eye by 0.6 to 0.7 mm. This "chromatic interval" or "linear chromatic aberration" is more than twice the thickness of the whole retina and is about ten times the whole length of the foveal cone outer segments.

It corresponds to 2.00D of lens power. This distance—in millimeters or diopters—has to be thought of as *the thickness of the retinal image*. In daytime vision, the yellow region (the brightest part of the *solar* spectrum) is focused in the layer of outer segments by the accommodation mechanism, and an emmetropic eye is 0.75D hypermetropic for λ760 nm (deep red) and is 1.25D myopic for λ390 nm (deep blue). In monochromatic illumination, visual acuity naturally deteriorates in proportion to the distance of the wavelength from the yellow locus of the spectrum, though it returns to normal if a lens is used to compensate for the "refractive error." In scotopic vision, the Purkinje shift of the peak brightness in the spectrum contributes 1.00D to the (roughly) 1.50D of "nocturnal myopia" to which all of us are subject. A shift of the spherical aberration caustic accounts for most of the rest.[22]

In white illuminations, most of the "thickness" and chromatic blurredness of the retinal image is caused by short-wave light, since the shorter wavelengths are the most greatly dispersed. The natural intraocular filters of the eye—the macular pigment, retinal capillary network, and yellow coloration of the adult lens—help to "thin" and sharpen the image. No demonstrable additional improvement in visual acuity is given by an *external* yellow goggle added to the filter density that nature has worked out.

Monochromatic illumination—plus a corrective lens—gives higher visual acuity than white illumination of even much higher intensity, for chromatic aberration is eliminated and the only blurredness of the retinal image is that resulting from diffraction, which of course cannot be eliminated by any means whatever.

The very oldest idea for a method of equalizing the intensities of two different colored lights was that of Celsius in 1735, who assumed that if two lights afforded equal visual acuity, they must be equal in brightness. (This idea is not entirely dead among illuminating engineers, even yet!) Actually, for all practical purposes visual acuity seems to be independent of wavelength. But, when visual acuity is *carefully* studied along an equal-brightness spectrum, with the "refractive error" from the position of the focus on the optic axis kept compensated, visual acuity rises slowly to a maximum in the yellow and slowly falls again toward the other end of the spectrum. The reason for this is not known, for conflicting evidence comes from various studies of intensity discrimination, flicker, and the like, with monochromatic illuminations, which might be expected to shed light on the matter.

Anatomical variations

Retinal position. Individual variation in the structure of the fovea and in the size of foveal cones probably accounts for a good part of the individual variation of visual acuity from eye to eye where the eyes seem otherwise identical.

The rapid drop in "acuity capability" of the retina as the image of a target falls off the fovea is well known. It is interesting that the fall-off of visual acuity does not precisely parallel either the variation in cones per square millimeter of retina or the square root of this number, although it is closer to the latter.[17] One would only expect this to be true if a one-to-one relationship between cone and vision locus were preserved in the periphery. This apparently is not the case. The fall-off of acuity at least to 15 degrees from the fovea is *not* the result of a gross increase of refractive error at the oblique incidence, as shown by Ferree and Rand.[18] Mandelbaum and Sloan[19] very nicely describe the fall-off in visual acuity as one tests into the retinal periphery. They relate their measurements to field and target illuminances.

Age. The effect of age is a controversial subject and probably involves several factors working at cross purposes. For example, the increased absorption of short-wave light in the media should be beneficial but may be masked by the increase in density of the lens.

Pigmentation. The pigmentation of the uveal tract is somehow related to visual acuity. Negroes have higher acuity than Caucasians and brunet Caucasians probably have slightly higher acuity than blonds. The same superiority of darker eyes is found also with respect to the absolute intensity threshold. *Scotopic* visual acuity, however, bears no relation to the intensity threshold or to photopic acuity, as the Navy slowly learned during World War II. Ability to see details in dim illumination cannot be predicted from any of the subject's other visual abilities, including "dark adaptability."

Pathological conditions—optical effects. The optical effects causing a reduction of visual acuity are manifold and will only be briefly mentioned.

Anything that causes even the slightest irregularity of the anterior surface of the cornea has a tremendous effect on the sharpness of the retinal image. Even small amounts of bullous keratopathy can markedly reduce visual acuity. In contrast, a small opacity within the cornea or lens that does not cause an irregularity of the overlying refracting surface will not appreciably affect acuity unless the opacity is very large. A patient's annoyance may stem from the opacity's ability to induce glare by scattering of light into the eye.

If a small posterior subcapsular cataract *excludes light from the retina,* of course, a decided drop of visual acuity will ensue; on the other hand, if the pupil is dilated so that light is able to reach the retina from around the opacity, sometimes surprising visual acuity is possible. I recall a prison guard who was totally incapacitated in bright daylight (when his pupil was small) because of a tiny subcapsular cataract. He had 20/20 vision in the decreased illumination of the refraction lane!

Nuclear sclerosis of the lens or water vacuoles in the central pupillary aperture of the lens may give rise to monocular diplopia or triplopia, since the affected areas act as independent "lenses" and focus light onto the retina separately from the image formed by the balance of the lens.

Experience

Every scientific investigator of the relationship of visual acuity to intensity, retinal topography, distance, or anything else has found that for days and weeks his experimental subjects gave better and better performances without any manipulation of the variable whose influence he proposed to study. There is no question but that visual acuity performance improves merely with *practice;* hence, it can be said to be trainable. Experimental subjects make improvements with time, that plot a typical sigmoid "learning curve"; until they show no *further* such improvement, the investigator does not bother to save the data they are producing.

In all sorts of commonplace situations, the amount of detail that one can make out—where resolution is an important factor or the only factor—shows itself to be profoundly affected by one's *experience.* Notoriously, an individual can do better on a Snellen chart if his native language is one that employs the Roman alphabet than if it is one that does not. An adult can read a line of printed matter when either the top or the bottom halves of all the letters are covered up, while a younger person may be baffled in the same situation. If a printed list of personal names is slowly brought toward a subject, he can "read" all of the given names from a distance at which he can perhaps make out not one of the surnames, each of which he has seen much less often in his life than he has seen each given name. Efforts are constantly being made to devise visual acuity charts with which past experience can have no influence upon performance. Such efforts are foredoomed to failure in the case of charts that could be successful with children and illiterates, for with such subjects one cannot hope to measure the "minimum separable" or even the "minimum legible" but only the "minimum cognoscible." These latter functions cannot be considered visual acuity at all, unless, with the French, we admit them as "secondary visual acuity."

"Psychic factors"

An additional factor that has great bearing on the "one-shot" performance of the subject in the clinical situation is a thing we must label "attention." In order to get maximum performance, the attention of the subject must not flag during the necessarily short test period. It is perhaps not surprising that the presentation of different letters to patients who have daily occasion to read commands attention better than a series of resolution targets or the Landolt C. This is certainly the experience of the great majority of clinicians.

An additional, even more intangible, factor is something that can be thought of as "mental set." Since the clinical situation usually involves a single sitting, it is much influenced by the mental attitude of the patient at the time of the examination. A recent emotional upset, antagonisms aroused by waiting-room experience, neurotic anticipation of eye disease, or simple fatigue can all cause errors in the clinical determination. These would not be a factor in the multiple trials of the laboratory situation. The physician must be sensitive to the existence of these possibilities and take measures against them when they are sensed. The simplest measure is a second visit on another day to recheck results.

The fact that visual acuities, both primary and secondary, improve with "training" is easily explained. But it has perennially been confused with the "cure" of refractive errors—in particular, myopia—by visual practice of "exercises," especially of the Bates' school. The extensive and careful studies in Baltimore and in St. Louis showed clearly that many myopes can "get more out of their blurred retinal images" if they try hard enough but that their improvement in visual acuity is not the result of any change of refractive status produced by the effort to see better, the practice with test charts, or the "exercises" taken.

SHOULD WE ABANDON THE SNELLEN CHART?

The Snellen chart—by which of course is meant the standard cardboard, block-letter wall chart *and* all its close relatives, whether projected line by line, or with a zoom system, or whatever, so long as the *targets* are Snellen letters (serifed or not) with a 5-unit height and a 1-unit stroke—has been cursed almost since the day it was born, loudly and often, as an unreliable test that measures everything *but* primary visual acuity (in particular, the patient's experience in reading); as a time-consumer that drags out the prescribing procedure uneconomically for a busy refractionist; as a patient-frightener; and as an unstandardized mess that varies so much when issued by one manufacturer or another that results with it on the same patient at different times and places cannot be compared at all. It has been officially disapproved on and off by organized ophthalmology since 1916. But almost everybody continues to use it in preference to Landolt ring charts, Ives visual acuity meters, and all the other much *younger* devices that measure *only* resolution but require 2 weeks' training of the observer.

Is "almost everybody" wrong? Should the Snellen chart be junked? To know what we *should* do about visual acuity testing—whether we proceed to *do* it or not—we need first to consider what it is that we really want to measure and whether the Snellen chart, or something else, measures this best.

The refractionist measures visual acuity only as a means to the end of "subjective refraction," and for this end he has no need of using enormous surrounds and intense illuminations. While, we believe, the practice of determining each patient's *maximum* visual acuity under optimal testing conditions is bound to spread and grow until it becomes considered "routine," the question of the desirability of this is not now before us, since it is irrelevant to the question as to what kind of *targets* and *charts* we should be using.

In our routine use of Snellen characters, we are making two assumptions: (1) that Snellen characters measure resolution acuity, and (2) that resolution acuity is a reliable criterion of all-around seeing ability. We may have to decide that both of these assumptions are incorrect. This would not necessarily mean however—as we shall see—that the Snellen chart should be abandoned in favor of something else.

Everyone agrees that "visual acuity" is *primary* visual acuity, or *resolution* acuity. Very few, indeed, of the letters on a Snellen chart constitute resolution targets at all. The L does not, nor does the T, D, F, A, O (unless it is compared with the C), P (unless it is compared directly with the F), V—ad nearly infinitum. A chart comprising only B's and E's, or one bearing only F's and P's or only O's and C's, could be a very fine primary acuity chart, but one might then just as well use Landolt rings with various orientations and be done with it. The one generally admitted great advantage of the Snellen chart—the familiarity of patients with its characters—would be lost.

For most of the Snellen letters, a visibility performance and/or a shape recognition performance is involved. The various letters, all at the same subtense, are not equal as tests of visibility or shape recognition. A few measure resolution or resolution *and* one or more additional functions. The chart as a whole, then, measures an inextricable complex of visual functions—not "visual acuity."

But is visual acuity a fair index of all-around seeing ability? We have no reason to think that it is. It has never been found, in laboratory investigations, that central visual acuity correlates highly with anything else—it does not even correlate highly with peripheral resolution in the same observer. Knowing the central photopic resolution acuity of an individual tells us nothing *else* about his general pattern-perceiving ability—his "visual acuity in the broadest sense" (into which even his color aptitude enters).

What the physician needs is a measure of the integrity of the dioptric system and fovea and its central nervous system connections. This measure must be incorporated into a test that can be executed with reliability in a finite time on an untrained subject who does not always have superior intellect. The test must be sensitive enough to detect 99% or better of disease at one sitting only. Despite the fact that the Snellen test measures a combination of factors, it fulfills these criteria. It is a highly useful tool.

We can say this, then: the Snellen chart does not measure resolution acuity, and we should not *want* to measure, and rely upon, resolution acuity. We can go on to say this: we want, or *should* want, to measure all-around seeing ability. The Snellen chart *comes closer* to measuring this than does any other kind of visual test. We can and should "keep" the Snellen chart. We should probably even try to find some way to work into it characters that would test vernier acuity and color aptitude also—and use the whole battery under scotopic as well as photopic illumination.

While our minds are on the Snellen chart, I want to "put in a plug" for the American Medical Association scale of "visual efficiency." It is wholly wrong to hang the label "20/40" on the visual performance of a patient and send him away thinking that his vision is only 50% as good as that of another man who is rated "20/20." This fact became evident so long ago in connection with medicolegal cases involving insurance and compensation for eye injuries that systems of rating *had* to be developed that expressed more fairly the percent deterioration of vision represented by a drop of Snellen chart "acuity" from 20/20 to some lower level of performance. "20/40" is *not* a fraction and should never be reduced to a decimal or otherwise treated like a fraction. The AMA scale of visual efficiency, printed on many cardboard Snellen charts, is probably not perfect; but our patients would be more fairly labeled—and much happier about their visual status—if we recorded their visual efficiencies and paid no attention whatever to pseudofractions with 20 or 6 as their "numerators." (In the AMA scale of visual efficiency, 20/40 would be 15% reduction from "normality," hence 85%.)

However, the numerators do have their use. Most charts used for acuity measurement are designed for 6 meters or 20 feet. Others, which are correspondingly reduced to subtend comparable visual angles, are certainly acceptable. Account, however, must be taken of the vergence of the charts when using them as fixation targets in the determination of refractive error; for example, if a reduced chart is used at 4 meters, you would require a spherical compensating correction of -0.25. The near test card designed for say 14 inches should be used at 14 inches, else the acuity notations on the chart cannot be used with any expectancy of accuracy.

The letter-size steps between lines on the standard Snellen chart are irregularly spaced (20/15 to 20/20 = 33% step; 20/20 to 20/25 = 25% step; 20/25 to 20/30 = 20% step; while 20/100 to 20/200 is a 100% step in letter size!). Although this arrangement may be acceptable for patients with good acuity, it is not satisfactory for evaluation of patients with *low* acuities. A chart constructed so that there is a geometrical progression of gradually enlarging letters between all lines was first suggested by Lancaster and recently constructed by Louise Sloan. The charts are commercially available and are very useful for work with patients requiring visual aids for poor vision.

We would also like to point here to the lack of standardization of two other parameters of acuity chart construction: these are the *space* separation between the individual letters on any given line and also the separation between adjacent lines. This difficulty can be found within individual charts as well as among charts of different manufacturers. The actual degree of inconsistency is truly surprising.

The importance of this variability lies in the influence of "crowding" of lines and letters on the acuity measurement itself. If the letters and lines lie too close together, the recorded acuity may be poorer than with single letters—perhaps because of an interaction of adjacent patches of retina (reflecting cortical interaction). This "crowding" phenomenon is especially prominent in patients with amblyopia, as has been so well documented by many strabismologists, hence the presence of the "variable acuity" of the amblyope, who may be measured in different testing rooms with different charts each time he is examined.

Thus, we would plead for a standardized chart, with the separation between lines and letters each made a certain percentage of the overall size of the letters of a given acuity line; the optimum percentages should be suggested by experts in this area, such as von Noorden or Flom.

OBJECTIVE METHODS

Much work has recently been done by Reinecke and Cogan[20] on the determination of visual acuity (here we are speaking of *resolution* acuity) in an objective way. The most practical way this can be done is by using the optokinetic nystagmus (OKN) response as an indicator. A test pattern is constructed of alternate black and white lines on a rotating drum that occupies almost the entire visual field. If an eye is able to resolve a given angular size stripe on the moving drum, it will be lured into following the stripes as they pass by, giving rise to the OKN movement, which then can be observed objectively. The measurements, when converted to minimum angle discriminated, show that the *objective* determination of acuity by the OKN gives a fairly reliable indication of a *minimum* Snellen acuity (determined *subjectively*); in other words, the Snellen acuity measurement is almost always higher.

The technique of analysis of visually evoked electrical cortical responses offers promise of giving us yet another tool for the objective determination of visual acuity. At the present time, however, it is strictly a research endeavor.

•   •   •

The foregoing treatise on the visual acuities represents an effort to tie together the dynamic psychophysics and physiology of this clinically important tool. I hope that now the big Snellen E is not all you recall when someone tosses the term "visual acuity" at you!

ACKNOWLEDGMENTS

I would like to acknowledge the help of Mrs. Gloria Haich and Mrs. Mabel Bass for typing and proofreading and of Miss Pat Hobson and the University of Florida Division of Photography for the illustrations.

REFERENCES

1. Weber, E. H.: Der Tatsinn und das Gemeingefühl. In Wagner, R., editor: Handwörterbuch der Physiologie, vol. III (part 2), Braunschweig, 1846, F. Vieweg & Sohn, pp. 481-588.
2. Fechner, G. T.: Elemente der Psychophysik, Leipzig, 1860, Breitkopf & Hertel; English translation by Adler, H. E.: Elements of psychophysics, vol. I, New York, 1966, Holt Reinhart & Winston, Inc.
3. Stevens, S. S.: The psychophysics of sensory function. In Rosenblith, W. A., editor: Sensory communication, Boston, 1961, MIT Press.

4. Hubel, D.: Transformation of information in the cat's visual system. In Gerard, R. W., and Duyff, J. W., editors: Information processing in the nervous system, International Congress Series 49, Amsterdam, 1964, Excerpta Medica Foundation.
5. Niven, J. I., and Brown, R. H.: Visual resolution as a function of intensity and exposure time, J. Opt. Soc. Amer. **34**:738, 1944.
6. Hartridge, H.: Visual acuity and the resolving power of the eye, J. Physiol. (London) **57**:52, 1922.
7. Shlaer, S.: The relation between visual acuity and illumination, J. Gen. Physiol. **21**:165, 1937.
8. Hendley, C. D.: The relation between visual acuity and brightness discrimination, J. Gen. Physiol. **31**:433, 1948.
9. O'Brien, B.: Vision and visual resolution in the central retina, J. Opt. Soc. Amer. **41**:882, 1951.
10. Toraldo di Francia, G.: Resolving power and information, J. Opt. Soc. Amer. **45**:497, 1955.
11. Riggs, L. A.: Visual acuity. In Graham, C. H., editor: Vision and visual perception, New York, 1966, John Wiley & Sons. pp. 321-349.
12. Westheimer, G.: Visual acuity, Ann. Rev. Psychol. **16**: 359, 1965.
13. Lit, A.: Visual acuity, Ann. Rev. Psychol. **19**:27, 1968.
14. Lythgoe, R. J.: The measurement of visual acuity, Med. Res. Counc. Spec. Rep. (London), vol. 173, 1932.
15. Brown, J. L.: Effect of different pre-adapting luminances on the resolution of visual detail during dark adaptation, J. Opt. Soc. Amer. **44**:48, 1954.
16. Cobb, P. W.: The influence of pupillary diameter on visual acuity, Amer. J. Physiol. **36**:335, 1915.
17. Ludvigh, E.: Extrafoveal visual acuity as measured with Snellen test letters, Amer. J. Opthal. **24**:303, 1941.
18. Ferree, C. E., and Rand, G.: The refractive conditions for the peripheral field of vision. In Physical Society of London: Report of a joint discussion on vision, Cambridge, 1933, Oxford University Press, pp. 244-262.
19. Mandelbaum, J., and Sloan, L. L.: Peripheral visual acuity, Amer. J. Ophthal. **30**:581, 1947.
20. Reinecke, R. D., and Cogan, D. G.: Standardization of objective visual acuity measurements, Arch. Ophthal. (Chicago) **60**:418, 1958.
21. Rubin, M. L., and Walls, G. L.: Studies in physiological optics, Springfield, Ill., 1965, Charles C Thomas, Publisher, pp. 89-91.
22. Rubin, M. L.: Optics for clinicians, Gainesville, Fla., 1971, Triad Scientific Publishers, p. 204.

CHAPTER *2* *Visual field*

MATTHEW NEWMAN

VISUAL ACUITY VERSUS VISUAL FIELD

A most misleading notion held by laymen and many ophthalmologists alike is the equation of "vision" or "visual function" with the visual acuity. Reduced to its purest example, the patient with cataracts and a visual acuity of 20/200 and the patient with a macular hole and a visual acuity of 20/200 both have a reduction in visual acuity to the same degree but have a marked difference in visual function. Then again, the patient with retinitis pigmentosa and a visual acuity of 20/20 has, nevertheless, a marked reduction in his visual function. The information required to understand the difference between the visual function of these three patients is the visual field test. The patient with the cataract has a marked reduction of both the visual acuity and the visual field; the patient with the macular hole has a marked reduction in his visual acuity but an otherwise perfectly normal visual field; the patient with retinitis pigmentosa may have a normal visual acuity but has a marked reduction in his visual field. We may say then that visual function equals visual acuity plus visual field. To understand the importance of the visual field examination, we must realize that two of the most basic visual tasks are detection and resolution and that the factors within the retina that enhance resolution tend to limit detection, and vice versa.

Resolution versus detection

Resolution depends upon the separation of detail and requires the analysis of the constituent parts of the input. Detection requires only that something be perceived and depends upon the pooling and summation of input.

The reciprocal nature of detection and resolution can be demonstrated simply (Figs. 2-1 and 2-2). If a ganglion cell requires 5X units of light for excitation and its receptor field is very small, then a small spot of light within that field containing 3X units will not be seen (Fig. 2-1). Increasing its size beyond the size of the receptor field without increasing its brightness will not enhance its detectability. It will not, of course, be perceived until the brightness is increased to 5X units. On the other hand, if a letter E is imaged on the retina with an overall brightness of 5X units in such a way that the arms fall on separate receptor fields and the spaces fall on still others, then the separateness of the detail of the arms and spaces of the E will be resolved because the stimulated

Threshold = 5x units light

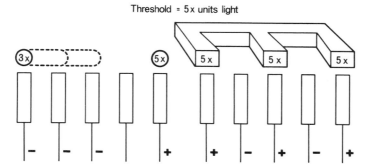

Fig. 2-1. Represented diagrammatically, if each rectangle represents a photoreceptor, which in this case feeds input into only one nerve fiber, there is no summation. Resolution of the E is good, but detection is poor since enlarging the spot size does not enhance its visibility.

Threshold = 5x units light

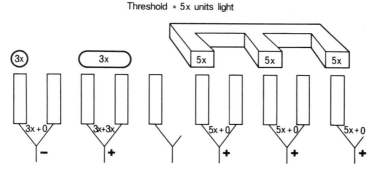

Fig. 2-2. When more than one photoreceptor feeds input into a single nerve fiber, there is summation and detection is enhanced but resolution declines.

ganglion cells are separated by unstimulated ones. Thus this arrangement with small receptor fields enhances resolution but not detection.

In Fig. 2-2 the ganglion cell with the same threshold requirement of 5X units of light now has a larger receptor field. In this arrangement, when the small spot of light containing 3X units is enlarged, the spot is detected even though the spot was not made brighter (Ricco's law). However, we see that the image of the E is no longer resolved because there is no unstimulated ganglion separating the stimulated ones. Instead of resolving the E, one detects a large spot of light—a blur. Thus, larger receptor fields enhance detection but limit resolution.

In perhaps an oversimplification, the retina is so organized that in the foveal area the photoreceptors appear to feed their input directly into individual ganglion cells and nerve fibers (Fig. 2-3). Such an arrangement, as we have seen, allows for the analysis of the input and the resolution of detail but does not permit summation. On the other hand, as we move centrifugally from the fovea, the number of photoreceptors feeding into each ganglion cell increases, allowing for more and more pooling of input—that is, enhanced detection but poor resolution capability.

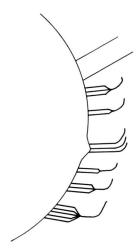

Fig. 2-3. The retina is so organized that there is minimal summation at the fovea and progressively more toward the periphery.

We can now perhaps better understand that in order to evaluate the visual function of the entire retina, we must devise two tests: a test of resolution and a test of detection. The visual acuity test is our clinical test of resolution and, as such, is nothing more than a test of the functional integrity of the foveomacular area, which in size constitutes only the central 1 to 5 degrees of the total field of vision. Perimetry is our test of detection and therefore is our test of the functional integrity of the remainder of the retina, which constitutes a total of approximately 125 degrees.

There are three basic variables in perimetry. As already suggested, the first and second are the size and brightness of the target. For any given size target, its detectability in peripheral extent is increased by increasing its brightness; for a target of given brightness or luminance, its detectability is enhanced by increasing its size. The third factor is luminance of background.

Detection

A target may be detected against a background in one of two ways: by either being dimmer than its surroundings or brighter. For dimmer targets, it has been shown that the smallest detectable visual angle can be produced by a fine dark line subtending an angle of 0.5 second of arc against a uniformly illuminated background.[1] Such a line produces a retinal image approximately one-thirtieth the diameter of a single foveal cone and creates a contrast of only 1% with the illumination of the surrounding cones—a dip in the level of retinal illumination that causes one or a set of cones to be differentially stimulated. Awareness of such a dimmer target is a function of the detection of the just-noticeable difference (JND) between two levels of illumination at adjacent photoreceptors and, for small targets, does not depend on its angular value. See Chapter 1.

The opposite, the detection of a small bright spot on a dark background, measures yet another retinal property not dependent on angular size. This is the liminal brightness increment (LBI) or, under the conditions of dark adaptation, the absolute threshold to light. The stars at night give the impression of a range of sizes. In actuality, the angular difference between the "largest" and "smallest" is inconsequential. A point source of light subtends only a few seconds of arc at the eye, but because of the effects of diffraction by the pupil, the retinal image has a minimum diameter of 1 minute 34 seconds. It is the difference in the total light emitted from each star and detected by the retina that accounts for the apparent difference in size. As the sky luminance changes from night to day, the "smaller" stars disappear first not because they are smaller but because they are dimmer and their contrast value is less. The critical factor in the detectability of a very small light spot or fine line on a dark background is not the angular size of the target but its luminance level and contrast value.

SUMMATION
Spatial summation

Ricco[2] determined that for a target stimulus larger than a point source, but with a diameter less than a given size (Ricco's area for any given retinal location), threshold was determined by a required number of effective quantum absorptions, which could be obtained either by increasing size and decreasing brightness, or vice versa, in the same proportions. Thus, for a small spot at threshold conditions, luminance (B) × area (A) gives a constant brightness or $B \times A = C$. Ricco's law appears to be a satisfying description for areas small enough to be served by a single ganglion cell (receptive field). Ricco's area represents complete spatial summation. As stimulus area increases beyond this to intermediate size, Piper's law $I \times \sqrt{A}$ takes over. Piper's area then represents incomplete summation. Beyond this, there is no summation. Threshold again becomes independent of area size and dependent only upon brightness. Spatial summation— the addition of subliminal stimuli to reach threshold excitation through the convergence of receptors onto visual neurons—increases with distance from the fovea and is greater for rod vision than for cone vision.[3]

Such areas have been found electrophysiologically in the cat to be approximately:

"Fovea"	20 minutes	
5 degrees	30 minutes	
20 degrees	60 minutes	Dark-adapted[4]
35 degrees	120 minutes	
"Fovea"	5 minutes	
Periphery	15 to 30 minutes	Light-adapted[5]

Some authors[6] have noted the equivalence in size between human summation estimates and the dendritic spread of particular types of ganglion cells. Furthermore, it is entirely possible that human spatial summation depends upon the activity of more than one overlapping retinal ganglion cell.

Effect of ametropic blur. In clinical perimetry, the effective retinal area of the target can be increased and the brightness reduced inadvertently, as a result of ametropic blur.[7] Because of the decreasing size of the receptive fields toward the

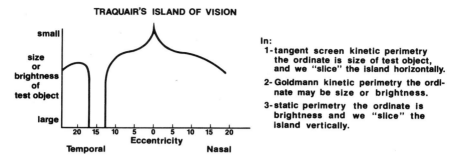

TRAQUAIR'S ISLAND OF VISION

In:
1 - tangent screen kinetic perimetry the ordinate is size of test object, and we "slice" the island horizontally.
2 - Goldmann kinetic perimetry the ordinate may be size or brightness.
3 - static perimetry the ordinate is brightness and we "slice" the island vertically.

Fig. 2-4. Traquair expressed the visual field as an "island of vision in a sea of blindness." Perimetry seeks to map the borders of this island with the kinetic method and the height of the island with the static method.

fovea, this factor is important only in the central 30-degree radius of the field. Patients should, therefore, wear their distance correction plus the accommodative requirement for the testing distance when this portion of the field is tested. Inasmuch as a spot of light (for example, the fixation target) is not an accommodative target, one should not rely upon the consistent supply of a specific amount of accommodation for the duration of the test. Failure to fully correct this factor can lead to significant errors or inconclusive patterns.

Effect of retinal eccentricity. Although the summative properties of the retina increase progressively toward the peripheral part of the retina,[8] there is nevertheless a gradual decline in sensitivity (increased threshold) to size and brightness peripherally, and the requirements for detection are greater (Fig. 2-4). This apparent contradiction occurs because there is a progressive decrease in receptor density from the paramacular toward the peripheral retina. Consequently, if we utilize Traquair's concept of the visual field as an island of vision in a sea of blindness,[9] and look at a cross section of this island in graphic form where the abscissa is the 0–180 degree meridian and the ordinate represents either the size or the brightness of the target, with the other being constant, then we see that the detecting ability of the retina is greatest at the point of fixation and declines irregularly toward the periphery.

Temporal summation

There is, in addition to spatial summation, temporal summation, which is governed by Bloch's law.[10] Just as with area, there is a critical duration of exposure below which the luminance and the time are reciprocally related. As exposure time is increased, a point is reached at which direct reciprocity between threshold and time breaks down; with further increases in duration the threshold becomes independent of time. This critical duration decreases as adapting luminance increases.[11] Although size of stimulus and retinal location is important, for clinical purposes temporal summation can be considered complete at 0.1 second.[3] Consequently in static perimetry, when exposure times of 1.0 second[12] are used, this factor can be ignored.

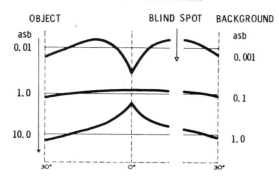

Fig. 2-5. Amount of light necessary for a spot of given size to be detectable at given distances from fixation at different levels of background luminance (states of retinal adaptation). The lower photopic curve reveals the greatest sensitivity at the fovea, with a gradual decline toward the periphery. The middle mesopic curve reveals the flat nature of the curve. A small scotoma can be easily magnified by kinetic perimetry under these conditions. The upper scotopic curve reveals the *relative* central scotoma. It is relative because the sensitivity of the fovea in absolute terms is still greater than under photopic conditions but it is much lower than the sensitivity of the parafoveal retina.

BACKGROUND LUMINANCE

Before considering the perimetric significance of this curve (Fig. 2-4) in greater detail, it is important to first discuss the importance of the third basic variable determining the detectability of a target—the brightness or luminance of the background. This variable is important for two reasons. First, the background luminance is the denominator in the contrast fraction. Simply stated, an object of given size and brightness has one detectability when viewed against a light background and quite another when viewed against a dark background. Second, the background luminance determines the state of adaptation. The retina in its complexity changes its functional interactions under different states of light and dark adaptation (Fig. 2-5).

Contrast

For target areas within the zones of complete and incomplete summation, the liminal brightness increment (B2−B1 or △B) required for threshold at a given retinal location varies with the luminance of the background (B1) in accordance with the Weber-Fechner curve. Above mesopic background levels (10 asb) the increase of △B with B is linear, both for central and for peripheral retinal locations. The constancy of the Weber fraction △B/B in the photopic range implies that the response of each retinal location is to a specific contrast value (△B/B) and not to an absolute luminance level. In photopic perimetry, since a particular contrast fraction △B/B is the brightness of a target against a background and it is this combination that determines the location of the isopter, changes in the absolute values of $\triangle B$ and B will not change the location of the isopter provided the fraction remains the same.

State of adaptation

The curve of Traquair's island of vision illustrated (Fig. 2-5) is the curve under photopic conditions. However, under mesopic and scotopic conditions the sensitivity curve not only rises (because less luminance is required for the same contrast) but changes its shape in such a way that there is a flattening of the macular peak in the mesopic range and an actual depression and relative scotoma in the scotopic range. As we shall see subsequently, the shape of the normal curve for the adapting or background luminance of the testing situation is particularly important for determining the significance of any scotoma elicited by kinetic perimetry.

Effect of pupil

It should be noted that the pupil plays a varying role under normal and pathological conditions in its effect on contrast. When we refer to luminance of test objects and backgrounds we refer generally to the conditions in object space. The physiological response, however, can only be to the light actually reaching the photoreceptors of the retina. The effective translation of light in the object space to the image space depends not only on the clarity of the media and the aberrations of the eye but on the size of the pupil, its effect on diffraction, and the Stiles-Crawford effect.

Changing the pupil size from a position of maximum dilation (9.0 mm) to extreme miosis (1.0 mm) will decrease the effective illumination of the retina by 1.5 log units. By way of comparison, this is the difference between the luminance of the brightest test target of the Goldmann perimeter (1,000 asb) and the standard background luminance of the bowl (31.5 asb). The effect of the pupil, however, is the same on both the luminance of the test object and that of the background, and the contrast value $\triangle B/B$ therefore remains the same. Thus, provided the effective retinal luminance remains above the mesopic range (where the Weber-Fechner curve is linear), the pupil size has very little influence on perimetric thresholds and the locations of isopters.

Under normal conditions with clear optic media, no significant difference can be demonstrated experimentally until one reaches the very small pupil sizes when diffraction affects the quality of the image.[1] Under conditions of reduced illumination, either because of the intentional use of mesopic or scotopic background levels or the clinical presence of cataractous changes in the lens, the effective retinal luminance (adapting luminance) is no longer within the range where the Weber-Fechner fraction is constant. Enlarging the pupil size will raise the adapting level and result in one contrast demand, whereas constricting the pupil will reduce the adapting level and result in a different contrast demand. If the contrast factor is fixed as with a perimetric test target, the location of the isopter will shift. Of course, the effects will be further complicated by the type of cataract and the image distortions it produces. The glaucoma patient with cataracts and using miotics gives the most frequently misinterpreted fields because of failure to understand these principles. Improvement or normalization of visual fields after radial iridectomy and/or cataract extraction may be nothing more than the effect of the adapting retinal luminance returning to the high mesopic or photopic range. In the perimetry of patients with cataracts, therefore, the pupils should be dilated and/or the level of background luminance raised.

TECHNIQUES
Tangent screen

Let us now examine the circumstances of tangent screen perimetry regarding these relationships. Under the usual conditions of testing, a flat black felt screen is used as the background upon which a flat or spherical white test object is placed. Both the test object and background are subject to the illumination present in the room. This may vary according to the conditions in any given office from ordinary daylight (subject to the variations of time and weather), to an overhead source of illumination such as a fluorescent room lamp that will illuminate the upper half of the screen more than the lower half, to some type of reduced illumination device. An attempt has been made in recent years toward some standardization of illumination through the use of the Gunkel illuminator. This device consists of a round fluorescent tube with a "high" and a "low" switch. It is arranged so that the patient's head is placed in the center of the illuminating source. When placed at 1 meter in the "low" position, the

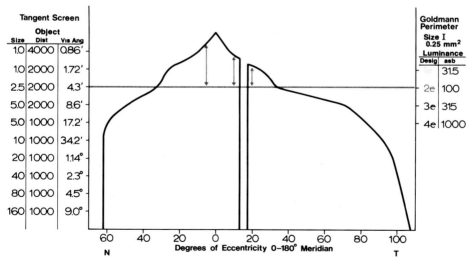

Fig. 2-6. A static perimetry curve through the 0- to 180-degree meridian of the right eye. The horizontal line represents one particular target stimulus level either tangent screen size (left) or Goldmann perimetry brightness (right). The intersection of the horizontal line with the curve locates the site of the isopter on the abscissa. The same target is then used to probe for scotomata and thus has variable effective stimulus value (see arrows), depending upon the proximity of the probing site to fixation or isopter location.

effective illumination at the screen is the same as it is when placed at 2 meters in the "high" position.

The background felt screen serves as a convenient place to put test objects and record isopters with pins or chalk. It also determines the state of adaptation of the retina, which we have already seen determines the threshold contrast demands across the visual field. However, with the Gunkel illuminator, the luminance level of the background is in the range of 1.0 asb, 1.5 log units below the background level of the Goldmann perimeter (31.5 asb) and well into the midmesopic range. For the above reasons, this can be a confusing range for clinical perimetry, especially in patients with opacities in the optic media. The Bausch and Lomb Ortho-Plot screen is lighter and when used with the Gunkel illuminator gives a background luminance of about 30 asb, which is comparable to the background level of the Goldmann perimeter.

Furthermore, the usual tangent screen test object serves as a visual stimulus only because of its ability to reflect the light falling upon its surface. The luminance depends on the type, color, and reflections of the material utilized. The reflectance also depends upon the cleanliness of the target. Using the same Gunkel illuminator and a clean target, the luminance is such that the contrast fraction is considerably suprathreshold for the central portions of the field. Consequently, only a field defect that is moderately far advanced will be discovered (Fig. 2-6). Attempts to overcome this resulted in reduced illumination targets such as colored test objects and the Lumiwand device.

Goldmann projection

The attempt to understand and control the three basic variables described before led to the development of Goldmann's projection perimeter.[13] A standard background illumination (31.5 asb) level was chosen in which the Weber-Fechner curve was linear. Since the size of the relative visual field is very sensitive to changes in the ratio $\triangle B/B$ but only little to changes in the absolute value of $\triangle B$ and B, a unit source of illumination was designed for both background and target so that any variations in voltage and bulb life would affect both and not appreciably alter contrast. Furthermore, by altering the illumination of the target alone and changing the contrast fraction $\triangle B/B$, isopters of various strengths could be obtained. This was a radical departure from the tangent screen perimetry of Bjerrum, which varied only the size of the target to obtain the different isopters.

In relating target size and luminance, it was found empirically that as the target area increased along one geometrical progression, the luminance had to decrease along another progression, also geometrical, so that visual field isopters could be maintained equal with targets of different sizes. Specifically, as the target size increased in area from approximately 0.25 to 1 to 4 to 16 to 64 mm^2, a factor of 0.6 log units, the drop in luminance required for relative constancy of the isopter was approximately 0.5 log unit—from 1,000 asb to 315 to 100 to 31.5. This relationship indicated incomplete summation with an overall constant of 0.84. However, it was further discovered, as might be expected from the foregoing, that with the target sizes and luminances in the relationship specified, the summation constant for the smaller targets was greater than 0.84 and for the larger targets less than 0.84 in the retinal areas close to the fovea. Toward the periphery there was less variance in summation between target sizes and the constant more closely approached 1. This meant that exact coincidence of isopters of "equivalent" test targets was not to be expected, but for the purposes of clinical perimetry, a constant summation coefficient of 0.84 could be assumed. The resulting instrument, using test object sizes and intensities as indicated before, has gained worldwide acceptance and has become the criterion by which other instruments are judged. By comparison, tangent screen perimetry is more primative and less exact. Other projection perimeters such as the Tübinger Perimeter of Harms are equally exact but are more expensive and cumbersome for use in clinical kinetic perimetry. The latter is, however, the instrument of choice for static perimetry.

Kinetic

Kinetic perimetry is conventional perimetry. It is the technique in which a target of given size and intensity is moved from the nonseeing toward the seeing portion of the field. The location in the visual field in which the target is detected is then marked as the threshold location for that particular stimulus. When all threshold locations for a particular test stimulus are connected, it forms an isopter, which then represents a line or zone of isosensitivity within the visual field.

Further study of the photopic sensitivity curve of the retina is useful for understanding the basis of static and kinetic perimetry.

In conventional kinetic perimetry, when we choose a test object of given size or brightness we are, in effect, picking a level on the ordinate of the graph and slicing the island horizontally (Fig. 2-6). The intersection of this level with the curve determines the location of the isopter. In tangent screen perimetry the ordinate level is test object size as indicated on the left; in Goldmann projection perimetry the ordinate level or variable is usually test object luminance as indicated on the right. In kinetic perimetry after the location of the isopter is determined, the area within the isopter is then probed with that target for scotomata. However, inspection of the *sloping* nature of the retinal sensitivity curve and the *level* nature of the target stimulus value demonstrates readily that the test object, though constant in size and intensity, is of variable *effective* stimulus value in searching for scotomata. For example, a scotoma near fixation would have to be much deeper in extent to be discovered than would a scotoma nearer the borders of the isopter.

Under mesopic and scotopic background conditions, as the sensitivity slope varies, so does the variable effective stimulus value of the target. Furthermore, a relative scotoma near the border of the isopter may not be elicited as a distinct scotoma but rather as a vague constriction of the isopter, a baring of the blind spot, or a breakthrough to the periphery, to cite a few well-known clinical examples (Fig. 2-7). It is important, therefore, when performing kinetic perimetry to verify such a vague finding by probing that area with the next larger or brighter target. The scotoma then may or may not be elicited, depending on

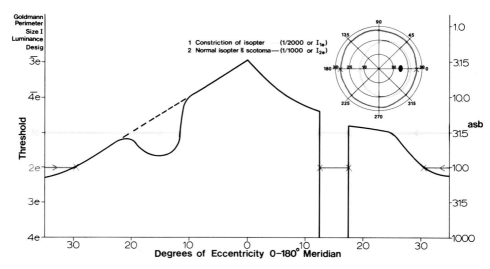

Fig. 2-7. Static perimetry curve through the 0- to 180-degree meridian of the right eye. Goldmann kinetic perimetric target I_{2e} will not elicit the scotoma at 15 degrees nasal. Target I_{1e} will not elicit a scotoma but a constricted isopter. On the temporal side the blind spot will be elicited by both targets. If the sensitivity level of the area temporal to the blind spot were depressed a few tenths of a log unit above the horizontal meridian but not below, a "baring of the blind spot" pattern would be elicted.

whether or not it is deep enough to reach the next target, stimulus, or isopter level. On the other hand, if one suspects a shallow paracentral scotoma, one can only expect to find it if one uses a very small or dim target, such as one that would yield an isopter of 5 to 10 degrees. In tangent screen perimetry, when reducing the size is no longer practical, such as with targets less than 1 mm, one often resorts to the use of colored targets, which is really a way of reducing its brightness and, hence, its detectability. With the Goldmann projection perimeter one is able to reduce the intensity of the target to sufficiently low levels without resorting to color to obtain isopters from 5 to 10 degrees.

Mapping scotomata

The discovery of scotomata within the visual field is an essential feature of the art and science of perimetry (Fig. 2-8). A scotoma is a nonseeing area within a seeing area. Once discovered, such scotomata must be subjected to quantitative analysis with larger and smaller test objects in order to determine the density or severity of the localized visual loss. Analysis of the slopes and borders of the scotoma often yields information of great importance regarding the severity of the offending lesion, the sites of activity and quiescence, and the direction of progression and/or regression. When the threshold locations of targets of varying stimulus value (isopters) are approximately the same, we refer to the border as steep or absolute. Such a border suggests a stationary or inactive lesion. When the isopter locations are spread out over a broad area, it indicates that the lesion has affected visual conduction to varying degrees and implies an active, progres-

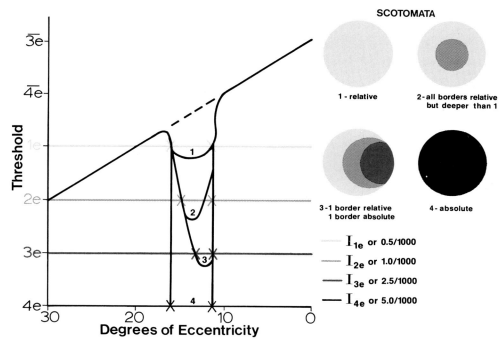

Fig. 2-8. Several types of scotomata and how they would appear by kinetic perimetry. Static perimetry would outline the exact contour and depth of the scotoma.

sive lesion. For example, an old chorioretinal scar with a focus of activity at one edge will produce an absolute scotoma with one relative border corresponding to the site of activity.

In kinetic perimetry the mapping of scotomata is subject to and may be distorted by the magnification effects of delayed patient reaction time and excessive speed of test target movement. This is especially true of small scotomata, of those close to fixation, and of nerve fiber bundle defects, which run in a relatively isosensitive direction. It is, therefore, often extremely difficult on followup examinations to know where a change is real or merely a testing artifact.

Static

The technique of static perimetry permits direct quantification of the defect and more accurate followup evaluation. Static perimetry is the technique in which a target of given size is placed in a stationary position within the visual field. The luminance threshold for that particular size target in that particular location is determined by raising the luminance of the target from subthreshold levels until it is just seen. In clinical practice, successive locations are usually tested linearly along a specific meridian or circularly at a given eccentricity from fixation.

Since the target is stationary within the field, neither the patient's reaction

Carl F. Shepard Memorial Library
Illinois College of Optometry 1033 Y

time nor the speed of test target movement is a significant factor. In static perimetry one slices the island vertically, that is, one measures the exact sensitivity of specific locations in the visual field (Fig. 2-9). Theoretically, one could do this by either increasing the size of the test object until it is just seen or by keeping the size constant and varying the brightness from subthreshold to threshold level. In actual practice, however, it is the latter method that is

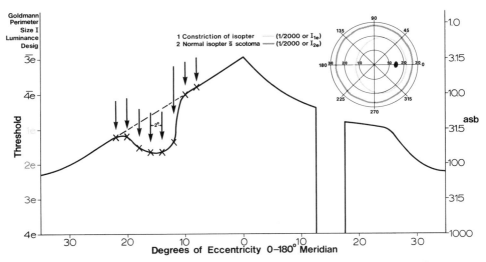

Fig. 2-9. The technique of static perimetry utilizes a target of a fixed size such as Goldmann target I in this case. The LBI of that target is determined at successive locations and reveals the exact extent of the scotoma.

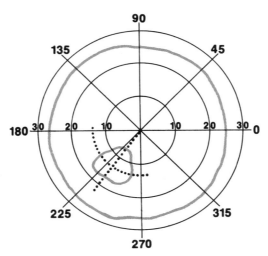

Fig. 2-10. A static perimetric cut may be taken through the scotoma along a meridian or at specific eccentricity from fixation. The successive testing locations in static perimetry may be in either a meridional or a circular direction, depending upon the clinical situation.

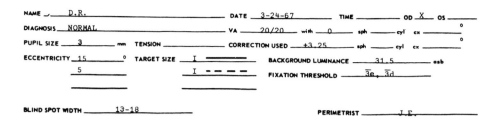

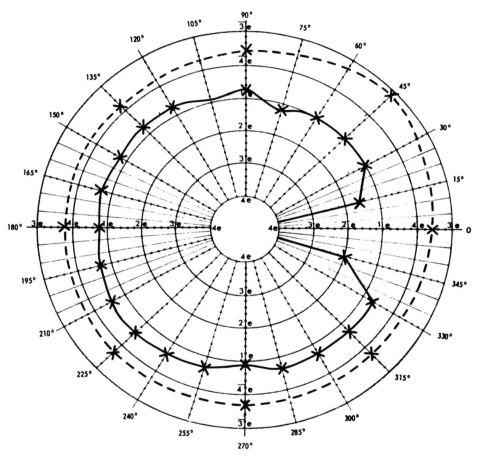

Fig. 2-11. When circular static perimetry is performed, it is more graphic to plot the data on a set of polar coordinates. The meridians correspond to the meridians of the kinetic field. Each meridional arm is the brightness ordinate of a conventional graph with the brightest level central and the dimmest level peripheral. Each plotted circle represents the sensitivity of a particular size target at a given eccentricity from fixation along periodic meridional intervals. A depression in the circle represents a scotoma. In the graph above, the inner plotted circle represents target size I at an eccentricity of 15 degrees. The depression corresponds to the blind spot.

used.[14,15] Static perimetry is not a substitute for kinetic perimetry but rather a complement and supplement to it. It is used to study a specific area of concern within the visual field. Whereas kinetic perimetry is ideal for qualitative diagnostic purposes, static perimetry is often employed for quantitative followup examinations to evaluate the natural course of a process or the response to therapy.

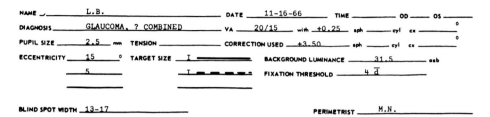

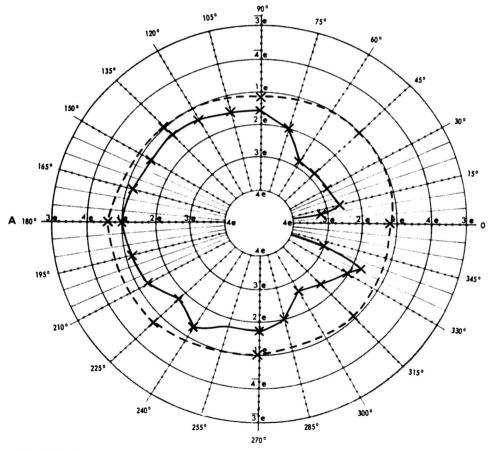

Fig. 2-12. Two examples of the circular static plot in glaucoma. **A** reveals the arcuate nature of the defect adjacent to the blind spot. **B** demonstrates the nasal step.

The sensitivity of a series of locations crossing the area of concern is usually plotted, and for methodical reasons such a series of points is usually chosen in a linear direction along a specific meridian or in a circular or arcuate direction at a specific eccentricity from fixation (Fig. 2-10). The curve illustrating Traquair's island of vision is in itself a meridional static curve along the 0–180 degree meridian (Fig. 2-4). When circular static perimetry is indicated, it is more

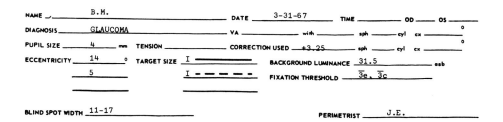

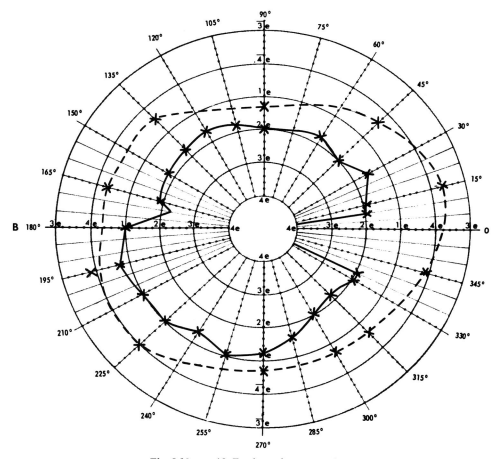

Fig. 2-12, cont'd. For legend see opposite page.

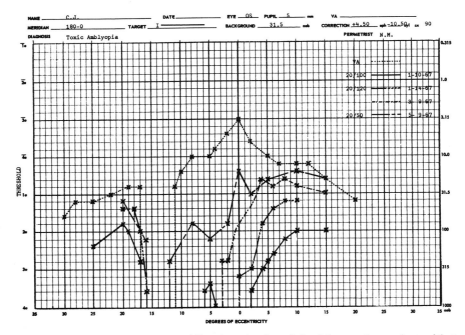

Fig. 2-13. Example of the use of a meridional static plot of the left eye of a patient with toxic amblyopia. Target size I was used. Dotted line represents the normal. Solid line represents the curve of sensitivity at the time of the initial examination. Other curves represent the levels of successive improvement.

convenient to plot the results in a circular direction on a set of polar coordinates where each meridian is the luminance ordinate of a conventional graph but corresponds in location to the meridians of the kinetic field (Fig. 2-11) and represents the threshold of the given eccentricity at that meridian.[12] Since points equidistant from fixation have approximately the same sensitivity, the normal curve of a circular plot should form a near-perfect circle. A scotoma would thus appear as a depression of the circle. A nerve fiber bundle defect, as in glaucoma, is one that follows a basically circular direction at the eccentricity of the blind spot. In the evaluation of glaucomatous field change, therefore, it is more practical to follow the patient with circular static perimetry at the eccentricity of the blind spot (Fig. 2-12). On the other hand, in macular and paramacular disease, when we are interested primarily in the relationship and proximity of the disease process to the fovea, it is more practical to follow the patient with meridional static perimetry (Fig. 2-13).

STATIONARY VERSUS MOVING STIMULI

Implied in the previous discussion is the assumption that kinetic and static perimetry measure the same function—retinal sensitivity to single targets that are just perceptibly brighter than their surroundings. Yet as a test of visual function, conventional perimetry, both kinetic and even static, must be accepted in perspective as being rudimentary. Functionally, we know that the optic nerve must signal various significant aspects of the visual field such as patterns of intensity, wavelength, specific contours, and movement. Hartline[16,17] demonstrated that movement of a visual pattern may be a more effective stimulus than the mere turning on and off of a light.

Lettvin and associates[18] demonstrated four different types of fibers in the optic nerve concerned with the movement of light and dark spots. When investigated further,[19] it was found that change of position within the receptive field was the true stimulus, with a maximum time interval required for this response to be obtained. Furthermore, directionally sensitive fields responsive to movements in specific directions have been described.

Clinically, a difference in response to moving and nonmoving stimuli was described as early as 1917, when Riddoch[20] described a category of patients with occipital lobe lesions who could see moving objects but not stationary ones. More recently, Fankhauser and Schmidt,[21] comparing kinetic and static perimetry, found that moving targets were perceived at a lower brightness in the peripheral field than the nonmoving ones, while in the center the reverse was true. Goldmann[13] found empirically that for conventional kinetic perimetry the optional speed of test target movement is 5 degrees per second.

LATERAL INHIBITION AND LATERAL ACTIVATION

It has been found[22] that in addition to the summative effects previously described, the spatial responsiveness of the light-adapted eye is characterized by excitatory and inhibitory effects. There are neurons, referred to as "on" units, which are activated by the stimulation of the center of their receptive fields but found to be inhibited by illumination of the periphery. Other neurons, referred to as "off" units, are inhibited by central illumination and found to be activated by peripheral illumination. These findings, originally discovered in the cat, were later confirmed in humans.[24] Studying the light-adapted receptive fields in the lateral geniculate body and striate cortex of the cat and monkey, Hubel and Weisel[25,26] found that the inhibitory and excitatory portion did not have to be concentric and circular but might be juxtaposed and rectangular. It was believed that the orientation of such receptive fields was important in the detection of moving spots. Furthermore, lateral inhibition and lateral activation enhance borders and contrast[27] and are thought responsible for such phenomena as Mach bands.[28] Aulhorn[29] demonstrated that the threshold LBI was elevated in the region of a bright band but not reduced in the region of a dark band. Furthermore, she found the converse true for discrimination of a decrement. This suggested that increment discriminations may be made by "on" units and decrement discriminations by "off" units. Inasmuch as clinical perimetric methods now available measure only increment thresholds, it might be well to investigate the effects of using perimetric test targets darker than the background.

Enoch's technique

Recently, Enoch and Sunga[30] have attempted to test the summation and inhibition properties of receptive fields clinically by expanding upon basic static

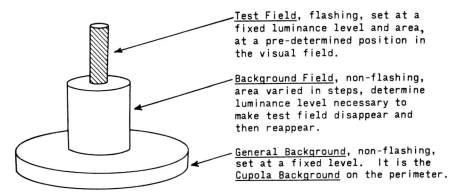

Test Field, flashing, set at a fixed luminance level and area, at a pre-determined position in the visual field.

Background Field, non-flashing, area varied in steps, determine luminance level necessary to make test field disappear and then reappear.

General Background, non-flashing, set at a fixed level. It is the Cupola Background on the perimeter.

Fig. 2-14. Schematic diagram of the three fields used in Enoch's method of clinically determining zones of summation and inhibition at different retinal locations. (From Enoch, J. M., and Sunga, R. N.: Docum. Ophthal. **26:**215, 1969.)

perimetric techniques. The Goldmann perimeter is used and the threshold for a small spot of standard Goldmann size (field I) is obtained against the conventional perimeter background (field III) luminance (31.5 asb) for any desired retinal location. The luminance of the test spot is increased by a fixed amount (1.0 log units), and an additional larger spot is projected on the perimeter cupula so that the first (field I) target appears in the center of the larger spot (field II) (Fig. 2-14). The large spot is made brighter until the smaller spot disappears, then dimmed until it reappears. Next, the size of field II is changed and once again the brightness is raised and lowered until field I disappears and then reappears (Fig. 2-15). The sizes of field II are also the same as Goldmann perimeter target sizes.

Enoch has found that in the normal eye, as field II is increased in area from size I through II to III, the luminance required to cause field I to disappear decreases. But as field II is further increased in size to IV and V, the luminance of field II required to "extinguish" field I progressively increases. The first is thought to be evidence of summation—as the area is increased, less luminance is required to produce the same effect, inhibition of field I. The second is believed to represent inhibition—as area is increased further, one passes from the central excitatory zone of the receptive field to the peripheral inhibitory zone and consequently more luminance is required to produce the same effect (Fig. 2-16). When larger than conventional sizes are used, no additional effect is seen, indicating that the inhibitory zone has a finite width.

Enoch has found that the receptive field, both excitatory and inhibitory zones, extends to the size of Goldmann target I (about 6 minutes) at the fovea, target III (about 25 minutes) at 5 degrees nasal to fixation, and between targets III and IV (37 minutes) at 10 degrees nasal, correlating well with experimental data referred to previously. In preliminary investigations of pathological cases, he has found that diseases of the outer retina do not alter the summative and inhibitory arms of the curve. Inner retinal diseases seem to have resulted in loss of the inhibitory limb of the curve. Optic nerve and pathway lesions have

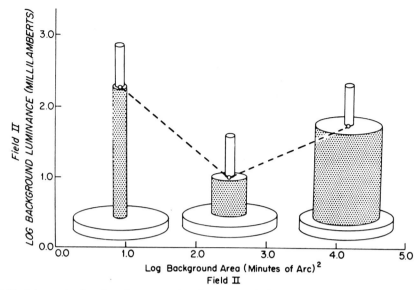

Fig. 2-15. Schematic drawing demonstrating Enoch's technique of determining summation and inhibition. The variables pertain only to field II. As the size of field II is increased, there is a drop in the luminance of field II required to extinguish field I (summation). As field II is further increased in size, more luminance of field II is required to extinguish field I (inhibition). (From Enoch, J. M., and Sunga, R. N.: Docum. Ophthal. **26**:215, 1969.)

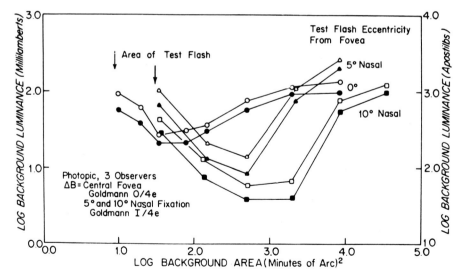

Fig. 2-16. Actual plot of data of Enoch's summation and inhibition functions at three different retinal locations. The open symbols represent background luminance levels needed to make the test flash (field I) just disappear; the filled symbols indicate measurements made when the test field just reappeared. The falling curve indicates summation; the rising curve indicates inhibition. Flattening of the curve reveals the boundary of the receptive field. (From Enoch, J. M., and Sunga, R. N.: Docum. Ophthal. **26**:215, 1969.)

shown no alteration of the curve. Although the results as yet are inconclusive, the technique is an ingenious one that should be pursued since it explores a parameter never before tested and opens a new dimension for clinical perimetry.

• • •

There is much room for improvement in perimetric techniques. Technical advances in electronics, computers, and automation have instigated new approaches to perimetric tests and have resulted in numerous clinical instruments, not all of which adhere to sound physiological principles. More important and more exciting, however, is the need for the ophthalmic clinician and the visual physiologist to cooperate in translating the scientific data into practical application for the good of the patient.

REFERENCES

1. Newman, M.: Visual acuity. In Moses, R. A., editor: Adler's physiology of the eye, St. Louis, 1970, The C. V. Mosby Co.
2. Ricco, A.: Relazione fra il minimo angolo visualee l'intensita luminosa, Ann. Ottal. **6**:373, 1877.
3. Barlow, H. B.: Temporal and spatial summation in human vision at different background intensities, J. Physiol. **141**:337, 1958.
4. Hallet, P. E., Marriott, F. H. C., and Rodger, F. C.: The relationships of visual threshold to retinal position and area, J. Physiol. **160**:364, 1962.
5. Glezer, V. D.: The receptive fields of the retina, Vision Res. **5**:497, 1965.
6. Bouman, M. A.: Absolute threshold conditions for visual perception, J. Opt. Soc. Amer. **45**:36, 1955.
7. Fankhauser, F., and Enoch, J. M.: The effects of blur upon perimetric thresholds, Arch. Ophthal. (Chicago) **86**:240, 1962.
8. Hallett, P. E.: Spatial summation, Vision Res. **3**:9, 1963.
9. Traquair, H. M.: An introduction to clinical perimetry, St. Louis, 1949, The C. V. Mosby Co.
10. Bloch, A. M.: Experiences sur la vision, Soc. Biol. Mém. (Paris) **37**:493, 1885.
11. Sperling, H. G., and Jolliffe, C. L.: Intensity-time relationship at threshold for spectral stimuli in human vision, J. Opthal. Soc. Amer. **55**:191, 1965.
12. Newman, M.: Modern techniques in perimetry, Int. Ophthal. Clin. **7**:949, 1967.
13. Goldmann, H.: Grundlagen exakter Perimetrie, Ophthalmologica **109**:5, 1945.
14. Harms, H.: Objektive perimetrie, Dresden, 1940, Zusammenkunf der Deutschen Ophthalmologeschen Gesellschaft.
15. Sloan, L. I.: Instruments and techniques for the clinical testing of the light sense, Arch. Ophthal. (Chicago) **21**:913, 1939.
16. Hartline, H. K.: The nerve messages in the fibers of the visual pathway, J. Opt. Soc. Amer. **30**:239, 1940.
17. Hartline, H. K.: Inhibitory interaction. In Straatsma, B. R., and others, editors: The retina: morphology, function, and clinical characteristics, Berkeley, 1969, University of California Press.
18. Lettvin, J. Y., and others: What the frog's eye tells the frog's brain, Proc. Inst. Radio. Engr. **47**:1940, 1959.
19. Grusser-Cornehls, U., Grusser, O.-J., and Bullock, T. E.: Unit responses in the frog's tectum to moving and non-moving visual stimuli, Science **141**:820, 1963.
20. Riddoch, G.: Dissociation of visual perceptions due to occipital injuries, Brain **40**:15, 1917.
21. Fankhauser, R., and Schmidt, T.: Die Optimalen Bedingungen fur die Untersuchung der Raumlichen Summation mit Stehender Reizmarke nach der Methode der Quantitativen Lichtsinnperimetrie, Ophthalmologica **139**:409, 1960.
22. Barlow, H. B., Fitzhugh, R., and Kuffler, S. W.: Change of organization in the receptive fields of the cat's retina during dark adaptation, J. Physiol. **137**:338, 1957.

23. Alpern, M., and David, H.: The additivity of contrast in the human eye, J. Gen. Physiol. **43:**109, 1959.
24. Kaplan, I. T., and Ripps, H.: Effect on visual threshold of light outside the test area, J. Exp. Psychol. **60:**284, 1960.
25. Hubel, D. H.: Single unit activity in lateral geniculate body and optic tract of unrestrained cats, J. Physiol. **150:**91, 1960.
26. Hubel, D. H., and Wiesel, T. N.: Receptive fields of single neurons in the cat's striate cortex, J. Physiol. **148:**574, 1959.
27. Alpern, M.: Metacontrast, J. Opt. Soc. Amer. **43:**648, 1952.
28. Graham, C. H.: Vision and visual perception, New York, 1965, John Wiley & Sons.
29. Aulhorn, E.: Psychophysische Gesetzmäsigkeiten des Normalen Sehens, Heidelberg, 1964, Zusammenkunf der Deutschen Ophthalmologischen Gesellschaft.
30. Enoch, J. M., and Sunga, R. N.: Development of quantitative perimetric tests, Docum. Ophthal. **26:**215, 1969.

PART II Visual adaptation

CHAPTER 3 *Rod vision*

MATHEW ALPERN

We see, fundamentally, because light quanta that reach the sensory or-ganelles of the retinal photoreceptors are absorbed there. The famous anatomist Max Schultze in 1866 detected two clearly different kinds of photoreceptors that we now know as rods and cones. Building upon the structure of a variety of abnormal functions in such diseases as total color blindness (monochromatism), Parinaud and von Kries independently developed the notion that the rods were used for seeing at night and the cones for seeing during the day. This idea—the duplicity theory—became one of the great gifts of nineteenth-century physi-ology to our modern views of retinal function. Cone vision permits color vision; rod vision is achromatic. This latter phrase means that rod vision is capable of differentiating one wavelength of light from another only on the basis of their respective intensities. It does not mean that rod vision is equally sensitive to the light independent of wavelength. In rods—as in cones—some wavelengths are much more effective in excitation than others. The curve showing, as a function of wavelength, the relative number of quanta necessary to produce some constant criterion response (say, the detection of fixed size and duration flash in the peripheral field in the fully dark-adapted eye in 50% of the exposures) is called the relative spectral sensitivity curve. The first way that rod vision differs from cone vision is in its relative spectral sensitivity curve (Fig. 3-1). For rods, blue-green light near 510 nm, for cones, yellow-green light near 560 nm, are by far more effective than all other wavelengths. More than 40 years before the discovery of rods and cones, the great Bohemian biologist J. E. Purkinje noted the change in the relative brightness of red and blue flowers in his garden as the sunlight gradually faded in twilight. This shift in spectral sensitivity of the eye in the transition from day vision to night vision (shown in Fig. 3-1) is now called the *Purkinje shift*. To anticipate a bit, the explanation for the Purkinje shift is quite straightforward. The photosensitive substances (whose absorption of light quanta excites the retina) contained in the cones have absorption maxima quite different from the substance contained in the rods.

A second way in which rods and cones differ is in their geographical distribu-tion in the retina; this is illustrated in Fig. 3-2. There are about 122 million rods and 6.5 million cones in the human retina. In the very center of the retina,

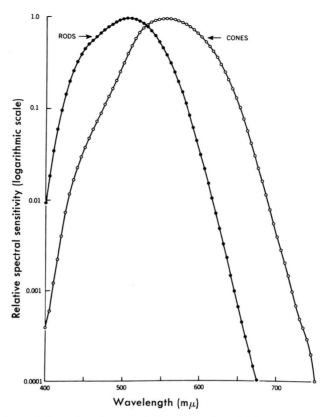

Fig. 3-1. Comparison of the rod and cone relative spectral sensitivity curves. The ordinate for each curve has the value relative to that of its peak. Note that the ordinate scale is logarithmic rather than linear. (From Alpern, M., Lawrence, M., and Wolsk, D.: Sensory processes, Belmont, California, 1967, Brooks/Cole Publishing Co.)

cone density is highest and there are no rods. Rod density, on the other hand, is highest about 15 degrees nasal to the fovea, that is, just on the other side of the blind spot. Although cones are found everywhere in the retina outside the blind spot, the relative scarcity of cones and the high rod density in the peripheral retina probably account for the fact that it is totally color-blind. The color vision is best in the center of the retina, where there are no rods and where the cones are most densely packed. At the very lowest light levels, the fovea may be at least a thousand-fold less sensitive than its immediately neighboring retina, which contains at least some rods. The French physicist Arago found on a dark night that a star that was invisible when directly fixed could sometimes be seen when he looked just slightly away from it (Arago's phenomenon).

A third way in which rods and cones differ is in the speed with which they recover sensitivity in the dark after a bright exposure. The nature of this process, dark adaptation, will be considered in detail shortly, so no more need be said about it here.

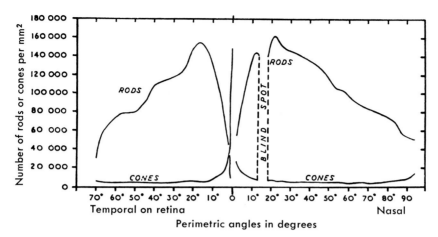

Fig. 3-2. Distribution of the rods and cones in the human retina. Instead of the retinal distances, Osterberg's values for the corresponding perimetric angles (eccentricity) are given. Although approximate only, especially at the higher angles, such values are more useful in practice than the distances in millimeters on the retina. Note that the distribution of rods and cones on the nasal side in and near the fovea is not given on this graph. It would be approximately the same as the distribution on the temporal side of the retina, which is seen on the left of the vertical line passing through 0 degrees on the angle scale. (From Pirenne, M. H.: Vision and the eye, ed. 2, London, 1967, Chapman & Hall Ltd.)

A final way in which rods and cones differ is in their sensitivity to the angle of incidence of the light quanta they absorb. The rods are quite insensitive to the direction of the incidence of the light, but the cones are much more sensitive to the light quanta passing through the center of the pupil than they are to the quanta passing through the pupil margin. This effect—the directional sensitivity of the retina—was discovered in 1933 by Stiles and Crawford[1] and is now known as the Stiles-Crawford effect.

Rods and cones, then, have quite different anatomical, physiological, physical, and (as we shall see) chemical properties. This duplex character of the human retina enormously increases its versatility. Cone vision is much more important in the complex spatial and color abstractions of the world required for modern life. But in the struggle of man to survive through centuries of long prehistoric nights, it was the exquisite sensitivity of the retinal rods to very small amounts of light that has played the more important part. It is this aspect of the duplex retina that concerns us in this chapter.

CHEMISTRY OF ROD VISION

To see must involve a method for converting visible light energy into nerve impulses, the only known means by which sensory end-organs communicate to the brain. The physical events involved in this transition are only poorly understood. Nerve impulses first appear in the retinal ganglion cells two synapses removed from the excited rods and cones. But the very first step in the process has yielded readily to elegant biochemical analysis, beginning with the discovery in 1876 of a complex purple-colored substance in the outer segments of retinal rods by Franz Boll and the rather monumental analysis of its physical and chemical properties shortly thereafter by Kühne at Heidelberg. It was seen in the human retina, in 1878 by Edward Nettleship. Kühne called this purple substance "sehpurpur," which was rendered "visual purple" by his translators Michael Foster and W. C. Ayres. It is now known as "rhodopsin."

Rhodopsin

Rhodopsin is a complex, conjugated protein representing about 35% of the dry weight of the rod outer segment. The remainder is essentially lipid. The rhodopsin molecule itself is a lipoprotein probably not very different from membrane lipoproteins. The best estimate of its molecular weight is 32,000, of which 18,000 to 21,000 is estimated to be the protein portion. The rhodopsin in the

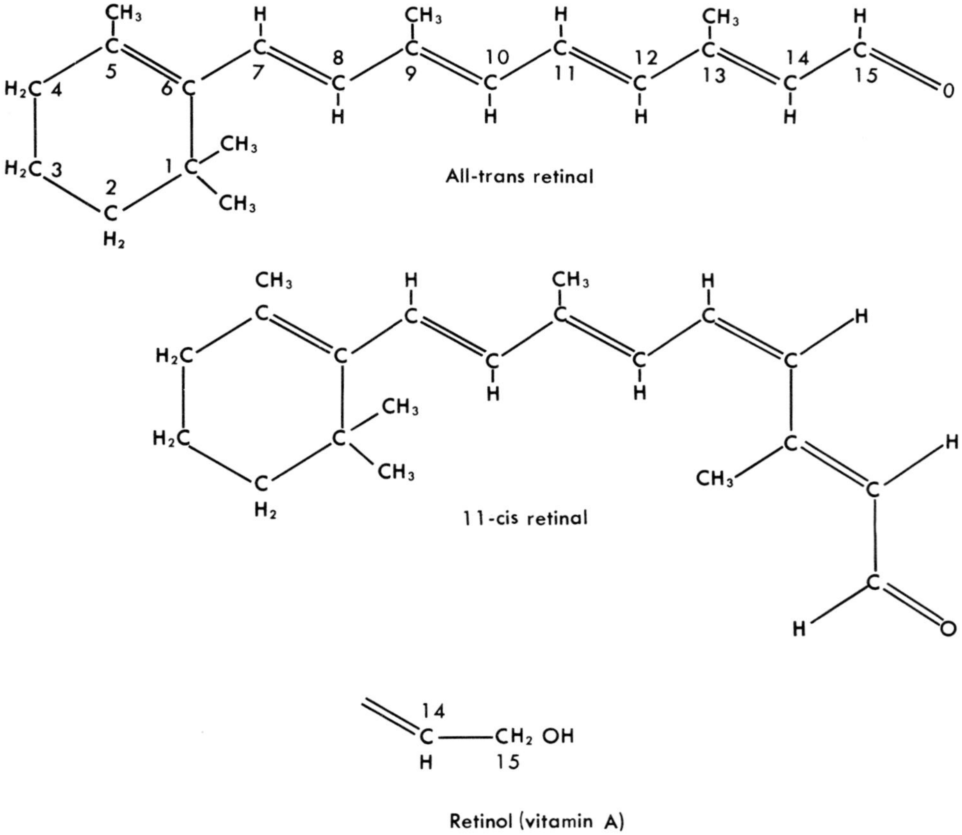

All-trans retinal

11-cis retinal

Retinol (vitamin A)

Fig. 3-3. The two stereoisomers of retinal concerned in vision. The all-trans form (top) is produced on bleaching but it is the 11-cis form (bottom) that combines with opsin to form rhodopsin.

outer segment is located in (or on) flat disks whose diameter approximates that of the outer segment stacked one on top of the next like a stack of poker chips. The rhodopsin molecule is composed of two essential components, the chromophore—whose chemistry has been extensively studied—and the protein, opsin, about which we are quite ignorant. On the disks the plane of the chromophore lies at right angles to the axis of the rod so that only light whose electric vector has a projection in this plane can be absorbed; and only the absorbed light can participate in a photochemical reaction (this is the Grotthuss-Draper law of photochemistry).

The chromophore of all known visual pigments is the aldehyde of a particular stereoisomer (the 11-cis isomer) of vitamin A. The structure of this derivative of vitamin A_1 is illustrated in Fig. 3-3.

This isomer (called 11-cis retinal) fits snugly into the protein—the opsin—and is joined to it in a way not yet fully understood. One idea is that this primary binding is a protonated Schiff base linkage producing an acid-N-retinylidene-opsin complex. The other is that it is an unprotonated Schiff base linkage. Each theory assumes additional binding sites along the chain. The absorption of a quantum of light produces photoisomerization; the chromophore becomes isomerized from the sterically hindered form into a long straight chain —all-trans retinal. Under physiological conditions, the only thing light does in vision is to isomerize the visual pigment chromophore from the 11-cis to the all-trans form. In the test tube a number of stages can be identified between the unbleached rhodopsin molecule and the end products: all-trans retinal (retinene) and opsin. These represent successive stages in the unfolding of the structure of the opsin revealing two sulfhydryl (SH) groups and one hydrogen (H+) binding group with pH about 6.6.

In the retina, because of the presence of the enzyme alcohol dehydrogenase +(DPN-H), the all-trans retinal is reduced to all-trans vitamin A (retinol).

Visual cycle

In order to regenerate rhodopsin from these photoproducts, two modifications are required. The vitamin A must be reoxidized to retinaldehyde (retinal), and either molecule or both must be exchanged for—or isomerized to—the 11-cis isomeric form. In the presence of opsin the 11-cis retinal immediately forms rhodopsin, yielding in the process a certain amount of energy. This energy is used to oxidize the retinol to form retinal. Thus, as long as free opsin and 11-cis retinal are available, the rhodopsin will continue to form. When all the free opsin has trapped its retinal, the process stops.

Several intermediaries have been uncovered in the stages of the unfolding of the rhodopsin molecule after the absorption of a quantum of light. After the very first change, the successive steps from one stage to the next are ordinary thermal reactions, so that by cooling the preparation to sufficiently low temperatures the reaction can be stopped at different points. In this way the various intermediaries have been identified. Whether each intermediary is on a direct line in the reaction or whether Lythgoe's transient orange—now thought to be metarhodopsin III ($\lambda_{max} = 465$) and indicator yellow—occurs as a side product

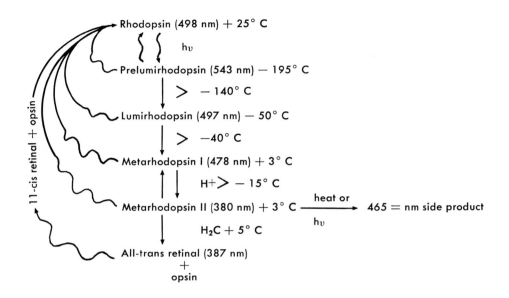

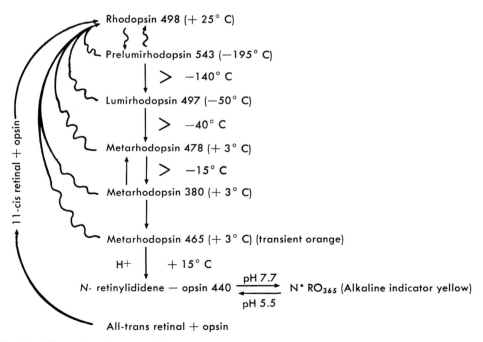

Fig. 3-4. Alternative schemes of the test tube bleaching of rhodopsin. At top is the orthodox view according to Matthews and associates (J. Gen. Physiol. 47:215, 1963). Below is a revised scheme according to Abrahamson and Ostroy (in Butler, J. A. V., and Huxley, H. E., editors: Progress in biophysics, vol. 17, New York, 1967, Pergamon Press, Inc.).

(or as an artifact) is still a matter of dispute. The alternative views are illustrated in Fig. 3-4.

In Fig. 3-4 ordinary thermal reactions are indicated by straight lines, photochemical reactions by a wavy line. The differences between the alternative schemes are probably not important insofar as the problem of visual excitation is concerned, because the time characteristics of these reactions are such that essential processes in seeing must have occurred prior to the reactions at which the alternative schemes in Fig. 3-4 differ.

However the differences between these views are resolved, it appears that all visual pigments behave in essentially the same way. The variants are mainly in the opsin. Cone visual pigments (iodopsin, for instance) can be synthesized with the 11-cis retinal from the rods and the opsin from iodopsin. Alternatively, 11-cis retinal from iodopsin mixed with rod opsin yields rhodopsin. Apparently the chromophore part of the molecule in these substances is freely interchangeable. Only one known variation in the chromophore part of the visual pigment molecule has been identified: vitamin A_2, which differs from ordinary vitamin A_1 only in that the junction of the second and third carbon atom in the ring is a double (rather than a single) bond. Vitamin A_2 pigments can be synthesized with opsin (protein) from vitamin A_1 rods and cones, and in general the λ_{max} of such pigments are shifted 20 to 30 nm toward longer wavelengths than that of their vitamin A_1 counterparts.

Pigments and vision

In what way do the biochemical events just described relate to vision? The answers to this question are largely unknown. There is a related and even more fundamental question, however, to which a quite unequivocal answer is possible. How do we know that rhodopsin is a visual pigment at all? Or, putting it another way, what is the evidence that the absorption of a light quantum by a molecule of rhodopsin is the first step in the process of vision? The answer comes from two related experiments—one physicochemical, the other psychophysical—on living human observers. The physicochemical experiment is straightforward enough: one measures the absorption spectrum of the rhodopsin in a suspension of human rod particles. The psychophysical experiment is the determination of the spectral sensitivity for rod vision: for each wave band in the visible spectrum one measures the minimum number of quanta required for threshold visibility of a flash presented in the peripheral visual field to the fully dark-adapted eye.

The results of this latter experiment must be corrected because, though quantum absorption occurs in the rod outer segment, we measure the amount of light emerging from the apparatus at the cornea. There is considerable loss of light in the ocular media that cannot contribute to vision. Unfortunately, these losses are not uniform throughout the spectrum. One major loss is absorption in the lens; this can be obviated by using aphakic subjects. Alternatively, we estimate the spectrum losses in the eye media by measurements made on enucleated eyes or on living eyes in which, because of one pathological condition or another, the back of the eye acts as a diffuse white reflector. Each method involves a number of untestable assumptions, but in each case the assumptions

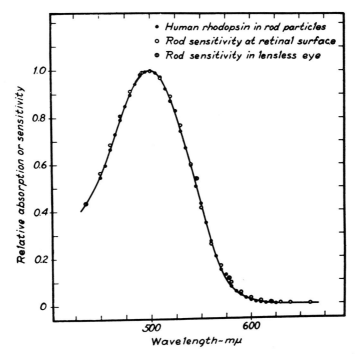

Fig. 3-5. The curve shows the agreement between the absorption spectrum of human rod particles (filled circles) and the spectral sensitivity of the dark-adapted peripheral retina in man. The open circles show the psychophysical result quantized and corrected for light losses in the eye media. The circles with the vertical line show similar results for aphakic observers. (From Wald, G., and Brown, P. K.: Science **127**:222, 1958.)

are quite different so that the close agreement found empirically lends support to the validity of the correction factor inferred by either method.

Fig. 3-5 shows the agreement between the absorption spectrum of rhodopsin in rod particles and the spectral sensitivity of rod vision of aphakic subjects as well as that of normal subjects after corrections have been made for losses in the eye media. The close agreement of all three sets of experiments is convincing evidence that rhodopsin absorption of light quanta initiates the sequence of physiological events culminating in rod vision.

A second parallel of a different, but closely related, sort can be drawn by observation of the kinetics of rhodopsin recovery following bleaching and comparing it to the recovery of rod sensitivity in the dark following adaptation to a bright light. This physicochemical experiment involved here, however, cannot be carried out in the test tube because we do not yet know enough about rhodopsin regeneration in the living eye to choose between a variety of possible alternative mechanisms (and there are almost certainly others not yet discovered) for converting, among other things, all-trans retinal (or retinol) to 11-cis retinal (or retinol). However, Rushton has developed a method for observing

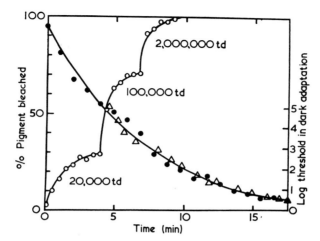

Fig. 3-6. White circles show the time course of rhodopsin bleaching by lights of three intensities in succession—20,000, 100,000, and 2,000,000 trolands, respectively. Black circles represent subsequent regeneration in the dark. Triangles show rod dark-adaptation curve (scale of rod threshold on right) using a special technique to measure rod thresholds above the threshold for cones. (From Rushton, W. A. H.: Invest. Ophthal. 5:233, 1966.)

the changes in the amount of human rhodopsin in the living eye, and this affords us the opportunity of measuring rhodopsin concentration directly at the place where it is functioning, that is, in the rods.* In Fig. 3-6 the open circles show the time course of rhodopsin bleaching by lights of three different intensities in succession—20,000, 100,000, and 2,000,000 trolands, respectively. The black circles in the same figure show the subsequent regeneration of rhodopsin in the dark. There is still a fair amount (about 5%) of pigment still unregenerated at the end of the experiment, that is, after 20 minutes in the dark. In the figure the triangles show the recovery of rod sensitivity as measured by the

---

*Rushton's method is conceptually simple (if technically enormously difficult). A mixture of two lights, a red and a green, is passed into the eye. Most of this light is lost by reflection at one or more surfaces of the ocular media or by absorption, but a very small fraction of the light, after passing twice through the retina, is reflected out of the pupil in the same way as the light from the ophthalmoscope. This light is focused onto a photomultiplier tube. The wavelengths of this mixture have been selected so that the green light is very strongly absorbed by the rhodopsin in the retina, but the red light is absorbed little, if at all, by it. The intensities of one of the two beams (say, the red) entering the eye can be attenuated by a wedge so that the proportion of red to green light emerging from the pupil and incident on the photomultiplier tube is identical (when the eye is fully dark-adapted). The eye is then exposed to a bright light that bleaches away the rhodopsin. This bleach will not affect the amount of red light emerging from the pupil because it is not absorbed by rhodopsin, but the green light is strongly absorbed by rhodopsin and, following the bleach, much more green light will emerge from the pupil than was the case for the dark-adapted eye. The balance of the two beams falling on the photomultiplier will be upset and the wedge in front of the red beam will have to be reduced to restore the balance. The amount of change in wedge transmittance necessary to restore a balance in the red-green mixture is a function of the amount of pigment bleached away.

intensity threshold for vision following a full bleach. The scale for this curve is on the right of the graph, where it is evident that what has been plotted is the logarithm of the threshold intensity. The fact that the same smooth curve fits both the chemical kinetics of rhodopsin resynthesis and the recovery of rod sensitivity of the same observer in the same part of the retina is a strong argument for the proposition that rhodopsin absorption by light quanta is the initial step in the process of rod vision.

The agreement illustrated in Fig. 3-6 points up a simple linear relation between the amount of rhodopsin bleached and the logarithm of threshold intensity for rod vision. The relation between these variables is mathematically quite simple. Unfortunately, however, unlike the relation between the absorption spectrum of rod particles and the scotopic spectral sensitivity curve illustrated in Fig. 3-5, this simple mathematical relation is not indicative of a simple physiological relation between rod threshold during dark adaptation and percentage of pigment bleached. This physiological relationship is, in fact, quite complex and will be discussed in some detail later. Nevertheless, the close parallels between the physical and psychophysical results shown in Figs. 3-5 and 3-6 can leave room for little, if any, doubt that rhodopsin absorption of light quanta is the sine qua non of rod vision.

ENERGY QUANTA AND VISION

What is the minimum number of quanta required for vision? This question was asked originally by Hecht, Shlaer, and Pirenne[2] in the United States and by Bouman and van der Velden[3] in Holland. Although there are some differences in the absolute estimates, the essential conclusion of both groups is the same. We will here consider the results of Hecht's group, which yield the more conservative estimate.

To optimize the sensitivity measurement, Hecht and his associates[2] made measurements of the number of quanta required for visibility of a flash of light under conditions selected to give most favorable rod sensitivity. These included the fully dark-adapted eye, testing the peripheral retina 20 degrees from the fovea, blue-green light $\lambda_{max} = 510$ nm, and very small area (10 minutes) and short duration (.001 second) of the test flash. Under such conditions the absolute threshold for flash detectability was found to be between 2.1 and 5.7×10^{-10} ergs at the cornea. These small energies represent between 54 and 148 quanta of blue-green light. This amount of light is deceptively large, however, when we consider that it has been measured at the cornea and that considerable losses must occur before absorption in the rhodopsin of the rods. For example, about 5% of it is reflected at the cornea and 50% absorbed in the lens. The best estimate (from the shape of absorption spectrum of rhodopsin) is that only between 5% and 20% of the light incident on the rods at this wavelength (the peak of the absorption spectrum) will be absorbed by its rhodopsin. Hecht, Shlaer, and Pirenne estimate that only about one-tenth of the light incident at the cornea participates in the visual process. Therefore it takes only between 5 and 14 quanta for vision under these circumstances. The area of the retina covered by this 10-minute test patch contains about 500 rods, so that if, say, 7 quanta are absorbed in this area, there is only a 4% probability that 2 quanta will be taken up by a single rod.

The inescapable conclusion is that the absorption of a single quantum of light, presumably by a single molecule of rhodopsin, is sufficient to excite a single retinal rod. Our rods approach the theoretical limit of any radiation detection devise. Of course, in a given excitation pool (see p. 76) several rods—the estimates vary among different authorities between 2 and 14—must be coincidently, or nearly coincidently, excited for vision to occur. This is necessary lest we see in the dark when there is no light, only the spontaneous thermal decomposition of an occasional rhodopsin molecule. But the rod itself is excited whenever its rhodopsin absorbs a single quantum of light.

DARK ADAPTATION

The characteristics of rod vision are clinically best studied by measuring how the peripheral retina recovers its sensitivity in the dark following full rhodopsin bleaching. To do this, one measures a dark-adaptation curve, that is, a curve showing how the reciprocal of the absolute threshold for vision changes with time (minutes) in the dark after the full bleach. The details of what is known of this process will be described shortly, but first some useful ways of measuring dark-adaptation curves will be described.

Apparatus for measuring dark-adaptation curve

In this section I will describe two different dark adaptometers. One of these is simple enough that it can be fashioned by any reasonable carpenter from readily available parts. The second can be purchased as a package from optical manufacturers.

The McLaughlin[4] adaptometer is shown in Fig. 3-7. An ordinary tungsten lamp is mounted in a lamp housing and the housing, in turn, in a light-tight box with a circular hole $5/16$ inch in diameter in the front. The test field is covered by two wedges rotated in opposite directions one over the other and so placed that the test field aperture is aligned with their upper intersection. Only one wedge of the pair (W) is shown in detail in Fig. 3-7. These wedges* were used in Kodak Color Densitometer Model 1. They are mounted in ring gears that can be rotated by the control (C).

The shutter (Sh), mounted also in front of the test field aperture, completes one rotation every 2 seconds and exposes the test field for any testing duration, say 0.1 second. A neutral filter (say, 0.3 density) can also be mounted in to cover the left half of the field, The subject's task is relatively simple then—to rotate C until the test is bright enough so that the right (but not the left) half of the field is just visible. If it is too dim, nothing is seen; if it is too bright, both half fields will be seen. Additional neutral and colored filters can be added as required in the filter holder (FH).

At the testing distance of 12 inches, the test subtends an angle of 1.5 de-

---

*Variable thickness, graphite suspension type, available from Eastman Kodak Company, Rochester, N. Y.

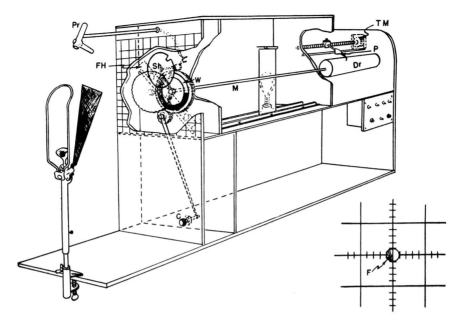

Fig. 3-7. Schematic drawing of continuous recording adaptometer. *Pr,* Fixation-point projector; *Sh,* rotating-disk shutter; *W,* neutral density optical wedge; *FH,* accessory filter holder; *C,* control knob; *M,* main shaft; *Dr,* recorder drum; *TM,* time movement; *P,* pen. Inset, lower right, shows the detail of the test stimulus; *F* is a low-density filter covering one-half of the disk-shaped test patch. The lines surrounding the test stimulus in the inset drawing are part of the grid that indicates position of test stimulus on the retina for any position of the fixation point. (After McLaughlin, S. C., Jr.: J. Opt. Soc. Amer. 44:312, 1954.)

grees. By projecting a red fixation dot with *Pr* to different parts of the front of the box, the observer's dark adaptation can be studied for different positions of the visual field within 29 degrees of the center. The foveal testing requires a special target.

The long shaft (*M*), which serves as an axis to the neutral wedge (*W*), performs a similar role for the drum (*D*). A piece of graph paper can be taped to the drum along which a recording pen (*P*) is made to write. A clock motor rotates the worm gear, which drives the pen motion parallel to the axis of the drum. Thus, after a bleaching light (not shown) has been extinguished, the observer sits in the dark adjusting the control (*C*), keeping the left half-field invisible and the right half-field visible. The rotation of the drum records the changes in wedge position, while the movements of the pen along the worm gear with time trace the minutes in the dark. The combination is an automatic record of threshold as a function of time in the dark after bleach, provided the light source energy and wedge densities for different positions are known. In fact, wedges of this kind are very nearly linear with density over most of their range so that under most conditions the pen traces a clear record of log threshold for the entire time in the dark.

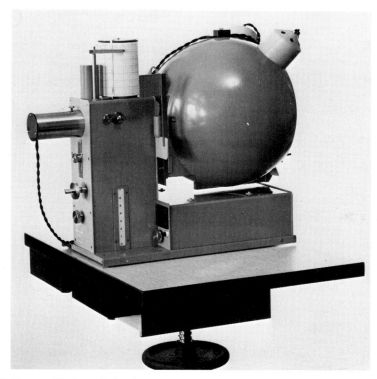

Fig. 3-8. Goldmann-Weekers dark adaptometer. (Courtesy Haag-Streit AG, Bern, Switzerland.)

Goldmann-Weekers dark adaptometer. A useful device for clinical evaluation of dark adaptation is the Goldmann-Weekers adaptometer.* It is more versatile in many ways than the instrument just described, but many of its advantages—such as the ability to measure the dark adaptation of the entire retina and the ability to measure dark adaptation objectively—have not yet been extensively exploited.

The apparatus is illustrated in Fig. 3-8. The device consists of a test target 11 degrees in diameter seen either directly on or 15 degrees below the red fixation point. When foveal function is tested, a red glass is used to filter the test beam. The intensity of the test pattern is controlled by a 7.0 density neutral wedge. The current to the lamp is held fixed and the target intensity measured with a meter accompanying the instrument. Several different targets are available including: a small 40-minute aperture, a Landolt broken ring, a black and white stripe either 100%, 20%, or 10% contrast, and an opal glass. The stripe or ring can be placed in different positions. There is a semiautomatic record ob-

*Manufactured by Haag-Streit AG, Bern, Switzerland; available in the United States through House of Vision Inc., Chicago, Ill.

tained; the examiner needs only to press a moving pin into the chart whenever a threshold is to be recorded. The apparatus contains a hemisphere 30 cm in diameter that gives a good light adaptation of the entire field. This same hemisphere is utilized for testing the sensitivity of the entire retina in the manner recommended by Jayle and Ourgaud.[5] For this application the entire hemisphere (evenly illuminated) is turned on and off at 1-second intervals and the threshold intensity, which just permits the patient to detect the intermittent exposures, is measured. The intensity of the light is varied with the wedge and measured with a meter supplied with the instrument.

All these test targets can be exposed intermittently (1 second on, 1 second off), continuously, or as a brief exposure at the examiner's volition. In general, however, the whole retina is tested by the intermittent exposures, the small targets by continuous exposure (although the intermittent exposure would probably be better employed for small targets also).

The dark adaptation can be recorded objectively with this device by replacing the hemisphere with a rotating plastic drum containing black and white stripes. The drum is illuminated by the test field light beam, intensity is varied by the wedge, and the plastic material gives even distribution of light in the drum. The eye movements are observed by luminous spots in a scleral contact lens placed on the patient's eye.

In using either of these devices there are handicaps limiting its laboratory, if not its clinical, application. In all dark-adaptation studies one is interested in retinal—rather than pupillary—function, and so it is best to control for fluctuation in pupil size. One easy way is to produce mydriasis by a mild topical drug, such as 1% tropicamide. The Goldmann-Weekers device does not readily permit testing a large number of different retinal areas individually or using the targets of a large number of different sizes (other than the 11-degree or 40-minute targets supplied). McLaughlin's device as described has only a single target size, the dimensions of the wedges being the upper limiting factor. (Changes in target size within rather narrow limits can be achieved without major modifications, however.) The Goldmann-Weekers adaptometer also does not easily permit exact fixation control for foveal testing, and the range of color filters available is small considering the increased potential flexibility that could accrue from a larger variety (say, an additional blue and green). Nonetheless, these devices have found wide clinical usefulness. When properly employed by knowledgeable examiners, they fill a definite role in diagnosis of retinal abnormalities.

Dark-adaptation curve

The dark-adaptation curve of the peripheral field (that is, of a part of the visual field in which vision is subserved by both cones and rods) is illustrated in Fig. 3-9. It shows the course of dark adaptation as measured by the minimum intensity of light visible at threshold in 110 normal persons. The points represent the single measurements made with two subjects yielding the highest and lowest values of the final threshold. The dotted area contains 80% of this population. For the first part of these curves (filled circles) the violet color of the test flash was clearly visible, but in the last part (unfilled circles) the flash ap-

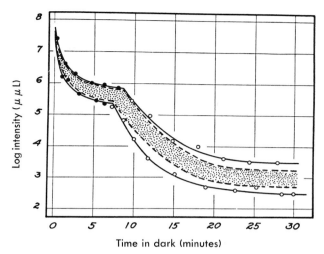

Fig. 3-9. The course of dark adaptation in 110 normal persons. The points represent single measurements made with two subjects yielding the highest and lowest values of the final threshold. The dotted area contains the results from 80% of this population. Note the cone adaptation marked with filled-in circles, the rod adaptation marked with unfilled circles, and the cone-rod transition time. (From Hecht, S., and Mandlebaum, J.: J.A.M.A. **112**:1910, 1939.)

peared colorless. There are several ways of proving that the filled circles represent the recovery of cone sensitivity, the open circles the recovery of rod sensitivity. The principal evidence is that if the action spectrum of the two curves is measured by using test flashes of different dominant wavelengths, the Purkinje shift appears, the filled circles have the action spectrum of cones, the open circles that of rods. Alternatively, the test flash may be put in through the edge of the pupil rather than, as is here the case, through the center; the cone part of the curve will then be correspondingly elevated but the rod curve remains unaltered, since the cones are directionally sensitive, the rods directionally insensitive, to the angle of incidence of the light (Stiles-Crawford effect). Finally, the recovery of the cone sensitivity goes hand in hand with regeneration of foveal cone visual pigments as measured with the retinal densitometer. Just as we have already seen, the rod sensitivity follows closely rhodopsin regeneration (see Fig. 3-6, p. 67).

The careful reader will note that the rod dark-adaptation curve shown in Fig. 3-6 covers a much wider range of intensities than the more usual curve shown in Fig. 3-9. This is because in making the measurements in Fig. 3-6 Rushton[6] took elaborate precautions to keep the cone threshold higher than that of the rods for a more extended period in the dark. Normally the rod threshold first appears lower than the cone threshold some 8 to 12 minutes in the dark after a full bleach and falls thereafter about 2.5 to 3.5 $\log_{10}$ units. This final recovery, representing 300- to 3,000-fold increase in rod sensitivity, is associated with a relatively trivial 8% increase in the amount of rhodopsin in the retina. This is because it is the *logarithm* of the sensitivity that increases linearly with the amount of rhodopsin (Fig. 3-6).

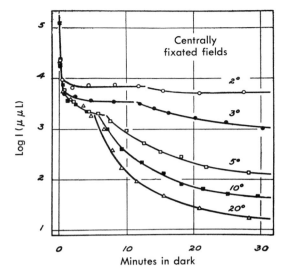

Fig. 3-10. The threshold during dark adaptation for centrally fixated areas of different sizes. The first and second portions of the dark-adaptation curves have been separated by a slight gap since it is uncertain whether the transition between them is sharp or rounded; most likely it is rounded. (From Hecht, S., Haig, C., and Wald, G.: J. Gen. Physiol. **19:**321, 1935.)

Photochemical events occur within the rod outer segments, and with a given amount of bleaching the rhodopsin kinetics are pretty much the same whether the rods containing them are part of a very small or a very large illuminated patch of retina. But the dark-adaptation curves obtained with different sizes of test targets are very different. This is shown by Fig. 3-10. Dark-adaptation curves were measured for a centrally-fixed test patch of various sizes, as labeled in the figure. The larger the test field, the more prominent is the rod part of the dark-adaptation curve and the greater the sensitivity after full dark adaptation. This improvement in sensitivity cannot merely result from photochemical events in individual rods, which, insofar as it can be determined, are very much the same whether the rods that contain them are near the fovea or at the edge of the retina. Fig. 3-11 proves that this increased sensitivity is not caused by an increase in the total number of receptors excited but by regional variation in rod sensitivity. In this experiment the 2-degree test patch was moved to different positions in the visual field as marked. Note that a 2-degree test patch 10 degrees from the fovea (Fig. 3-11) has about the same dark-adaptation characteristics as a 20-degree circular test patch centrally fixed (Fig. 3-10). In the latter case, apparently the most sensitive retinal area excited by the test patch determines the sensitivity.

Rushton and Westheimer[7] provided an even more unequivocal experimental proof that it is not only the chemical events in individual rods that determine their sensitivity. They measured dark adaptation curves for two fields, one above, the other below the fixation point. The parts of the retina corresponding

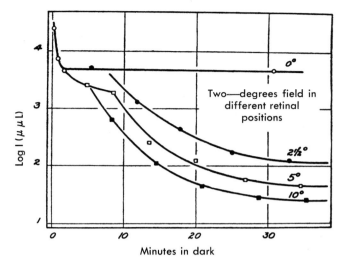

Fig. 3-11. Dark adaptation as measured with a 2-degree field placed at different distances from the center. Compare this with Fig. 3-10 for centrally fixated fields of different size. (From Hecht, S., Haig, C., and Wald, G.: J. Gen. Physiol. **19**:321, 1935.)

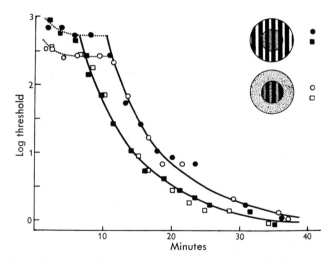

Fig. 3-12. Dark-adaptation curves showing rod and cone branches. Circles after mean bleaching flash of about 7 log sec; squares after bleaching with additional 0.5 density filter interposed. Insets: Large circle shows bleaching field with grating or uniform light distribution; small circle shows test flash with light distribution reversed. Bright and dark bars of grating each subtend 0.5 degree. (From Rushton, W. A. H., and Westheimer, G.: J. Physiol. **164**:318, 1962.)

to the two fields were both bleached by the same amount of light—the lower having uniform distribution throughout the field, the upper being distributed in a series of black and white bars. Following bleaching by a very brief flash, the dark-adaptation curves were measured for the two fields—the lower for a test of black and white bars, the upper for a uniform field equated so that it contained the same total light flux. The open squares in Fig. 3-12 show the measurements on the lower retinal area, the filled squares on the upper retinal area. The two curves go hand in hand even though the upper field (black and white bars in the bleach, uniform field in the test) contains many rods that were bleached little, if at all, while all of the rods in the lower field (uniform bleach, black and white bars for test) were bleached away. This result suggests that the state of adaptation of neighboring rods has a pronounced effect on the threshold of even those rods whose rhodopsin was bleached little, if at all. This interpretation is true provided only that the bleaching light was not so bright that even the rods viewing the black bars of the bleaching field were not fully bleached. This possibility is excluded by the experiment illustrated by the circles, which is an exact duplication of the experiments described previously except that the bleaching lights are three times as bright.

This interpretation applies to the rod curves in Fig. 3-12 but not to those for cones. This is because the frequency of repetition of the black and white bars in the bleaching and test fields was so low that it was at the upper limit of the boundary of the "summation pool" for rod vision (about ½ degree for the subject shown in this figure). This is considerably larger than the upper limit for cone vision, so that in this case the cones in the region of the bleach field excited by the black bars determine threshold. This accounts for the fact that in Fig. 3-12 in the cone branches of the curves the symbols have changed partners.*

We have outlined in some detail some of the characteristics of the normal dark-adaptation curve and the way it is altered by certain stimulus variables. Of course, there are a great many of these, and here we can only summarize briefly the important ones. These include first and foremost the intensity and duration of prior light adaptation. The results of one such experiment are illustrated in Fig. 3-13, which shows the recovery of sensitivity of the 30-degree temporal visual field to a 5-degree test flash of violet light after 2 minutes of light adaptation to lights of various intensities.† As before (Figs. 3-10 and 3-11) the points defined by the filled symbols show the region where the violet test flash appears colored and de-

---

*The bleaching and testing conditions are equated in this experiment by assuming that the retina integrates light over the whole summation pool. For rod vision the assumption is valid, and it is the total light flux emerging through the black and white field that must be equated to the uniform field. This requires a density 0.4 to be used in the uniform field to make it equally effective for rod vision as the black and white striped field. For cone vision this is no longer true, and in this case only the light emerging through the white bars in the black and white test field is relevant for cone threshold. The slide containing the black and white bars used in the test (as well as the bleaching) field had a density of 0.1 in the white part of the slide, and so (since a correction of 0.4 was actually used) the measurements for cone vision are 0.3 $\log_{10}$ units higher when tested by the uniform field than by the black and white striped field.

†The unit used to define the adaptation intensity, the parameter in this figure, is photons. This is the intensity of retinal illuminance obtained by multiplying the luminance of the field (cd/m²) by the area (in mm²) of the artificial pupil—or limiting aperture—in this case 1 mm². Since photon is used synonymously with light quanta, we now apply the name *troland* to such units, after the man who invented it.

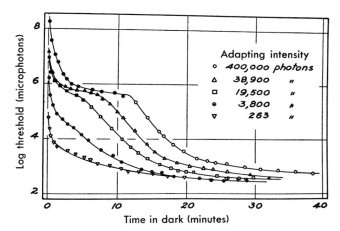

Fig. 3-13. The course of dark adaptation as measured with violet light following different degrees of light adaptation. The filled-in symbols indicate that a violet color was apparent at the threshold, while the empty symbols indicate that the threshold was colorless. (From Hecht, S., Haig, C., and Chase, A. M.: J. Gen. Physiol. **20:**831, 1937.)

fine the cone adaptation; the unfilled symbols illustrate recovery of sensitivity of rods. Look, for the moment, at only the final recovery of rod sensitivity from a position on the curves 100 times (that is, 2 $\log_{10}$ units above) the fully dark-adapted value. Clearly, recovery from this point is much quicker if the prior light adaptation has been very weak than if it has been very bright. This could not be the case if threshold depended only on rhodopsin concentration in the rods on the basis of any simple scheme of pigment resynthesis. While various attempts have been made to complicate the way rhodopsin is presumed to resynthesize in vivo to fit these observed facts, it is now clear that these different rates of recovery of threshold do not necessarily directly reflect differences in pigment resynthesis.

Other factors affecting the rate of recovery of dark sensitivity can, of course, include anything that influences how much light reaches the retina. One relatively trivial consideration is the size of the pupil. The pupil is small in bright light and very wide in the dark. After a very bright bleach the pupil does not immediately assume its fully dark-adapted mydriasis. The process, in fact, is as slow as the recovery of retinal sensitivity.[8] While this is of some theoretical interest, it also has a very practical consequence. If we are interested in only how the retinal sensitivity recovers, we can be led quantitatively astray by artifacts from pupil size fluctuation unless an adaptometer is designed so that the amount of light reaching the retina is not influenced by the size of the patient's own natural pupil. Neither of the adaptometers described in this chapter fulfills this requirement, however. When using them for our studies, therefore, it is best to obviate this source of error by fixing the patient's pupil at a fully dilated position by topical mydriatic drops, as we have already seen.

A number of retinal and general pathological conditions influence dark adaptation, and these will be summarized in Chapter 4. Vitamin A deficiency is said to elevate both rod and cone thresholds but not the time of the rod-cone transition. On the other hand, cirrhosis of the liver is thought to elevate all three. More recent evidence on rats[9] suggests that the evidence of rhodopsin losses only begins to occur after the liver vitamin A store has been appreciably depleted. Anoxia, hypoxia, hyperventilation, and respiratory acidosis are all known to influence absolute threshold of vision. Retinal diseases—such as retinitis pigmentosa, Oguchi's disease, choroideremia, stationary night blindness—and neuro-ophthalmological disorders—such as hysterical amblyopia—have been reported to affect rod dark-adaptation curves appreciably.

LIGHT ADAPTATION

We have talked above about the transition from light to dark. We saw that a fully bleached retina leaves traces that last for more than 30 minutes in the dark. On the other hand, when we make the change in the opposite direction the equilibrium sensitivity is reached much more quickly. This is also evident in the rhodopsin kinetics shown in Fig. 3-6. The changes in light adaptation can be studied by making measurements of sensitivity as a function of background intensity. At very dim backgrounds the intensity required for threshold differs little or not at all from the value in total darkness. As the background intensity rises so does the threshold, and at moderate levels the threshold intensity approaches some constant fraction of the background (so-called Weber's law). Interestingly enough, the curve that depicts the relation between the threshold and the background intensities for light adaptation closely parallel the curve for dark adaptation. For example, the rod dark-adaptation curves in Fig. 3-10 change shape considerably with increase in size of the test field. In a similar way the light-adaptation curves also change shape with diameter of the test object. This similarity was first observed by Crawford,[10] whose results are shown in Fig. 3-14. The left-hand curves are ordinary dark-adaptation curves for test objects of different sizes such as we have already discussed. (The curves are here plotted as a function of log time instead of linear time, but this difference need not trouble us.) The right-hand curves are light-adaptation curves showing threshold as a function of background intensity for the same size of test targets. Crawford[10] adopted the concept of equivalent background, that is, the background intensity that would be required to produce the same threshold as that obtained at a given moment in the dark. He could then plot a dark-adaptation curve, not as heretofore by showing the change in threshold with time in the dark but by showing the change in equivalent background with time in the dark. When he did this for test objects of different sizes he found the curve was always the same: equivalent background was invariant with test object size. At any moment in the dark the background intensity required to produce an equivalent elevation in the threshold as the one actually measured was always the same independent of test target size. The reader may want to make a careful analysis of the results shown in Fig. 3-14 to convince himself that this is exactly true. Thus, it is the logarithm of the equivalent background that is uniquely related (and linearly) with the concentration of rhodopsin regenerated in the rods.

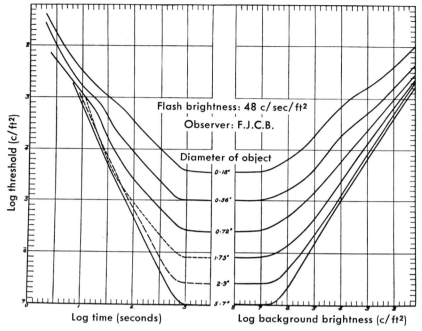

Fig. 3-14. On the left are dark-adaptation curves for test flashes of different angular substances, on the right light adaptation on real backgrounds for the same test targets. When the equivalent background of the bleach is plotted as a function of time in the dark, the results for the different target sizes all superimpose. (From Crawford, B. H.: Proc. Roy. Soc. [Biol.] **134:**283, 1947.)

THEORY OF ADAPTATION

We are led in this way to the most intriguing question in modern retinal physiology: what is the means by which the retina controls its sensitivity so that it is capable of responding over a very wide range of intensities to very small increments of light? We have already seen that at the lower limits the retina approaches the theoretical limit of any radiation detector. The other extreme—the background intensity so bright that the retina starts to burn—is over 10^{13} times higher than the absolute threshold. Clearly, we see by detecting very small increments and decrements in the light over this wide range. How? In the early days of the present century it was often suggested that this characteristic was the result of the absorption properties of the rhodopsin in the rods and those of the comparable cone pigments. The simplest photochemical ideas led to a linear relation between fraction of pigment bleached and threshold. This linear relationship was, in fact, postulated by Hecht[11] for light adaptation and hinted at by his student Wald[12] for both light and dark adaptation. However, this idea cannot be experimentally confirmed, as was evidenced as long ago as 1939 when Granit and his associates[13] showed that in frogs and cats after full rhodopsin bleach there was not an elevation of ERG threshold by a factor of 2 when 50%

of the rhodopsin was resynthesized. In fact, the ERG only begins to appear at this stage in rhodopsin resynthesis.

When it was possible to measure rhodopsin in living eyes, it was clear that a rhodopsin regeneration of 92% occurs at the transition from cone threshold to the first rod threshold (the "kink") in the dark-adaptation curve at the moment when rod threshold is at least 1,000 times its final dark value. Rushton[14] showed the linear relation between rhodopsin concentration and log threshold in man (Fig. 3-6), and this was also found in vitamin A–deficient, as well as in light- and dark-adapted, albino rats by Dowling and Wald.[9] The meaning of this relationship is far from well understood. Apparently each rod signals the amount of rhodopsin regenerating in its outer segment to an "excitation pool," and it is the state of excitation of all the rods in the pool that determines the threshold. Rushton and Westheimer[7] showed that the threshold in unbleached rods is elevated just as strongly as is that in their bleached neighbors, as we have already seen. Apparently the log of the equivalent background of bleaching is some linear function of rhodopsin regeneration. But it is the state of adaptation of the pool that determines threshold, though the signals (as to extent of rhodopsin bleaching) from the rods in the pool play an important part. How is this brought about?

Rushton[15] has built a very elegant model of the excitation pool based upon the theory of the generator potential in the limulus retinula cell developed by Fuortes and Hodgkin.[16] Rushton's basic idea is that a large number of rods feed into a common pool. The excitation pool is analogous to the automatic gain control of an amplification device. The input to the device (from the rods) is linearly dependent upon the light intensity. The output of this device varies roughly as the logarithm of the light intensity. This output has two destinations: (1) to the brain to signal the light and its intensity and (2) back into the automatic gain control device to regulate the sensitivity of the pool.

The linear relation between the amount of rhodopsin regenerated and the log sensitivity according to this model is brought about by the equivalent background of bleaching. The signals from the rods, indicating the state of rhodopsin resynthesis, are fed into the pool; this governs the pool's sensitivity. How does it come that the equivalent background of bleaching is itself not visible? This question was studied by Barlow and Sparrock[17] who point out that the after-effects of a bright bleach are stabilized on the retina so that eye movements do not displace it with respect to the retinal mosaic. After-effects of bleaching are, of course, visible as positive after-images, but they usually are not visible for the 30 minutes that the threshold is elevated during dark adaptation. Barlow and Sparrock showed that this was because the positive after-image, a stabilized image, fades—as all stabilized images do. They matched the brightness of the after-image with the brightness of a stabilized image in an adjacent part of the retina, and in this way they could trace effects of the after-image for more than 30 minutes in the dark. Moreover, the threshold for a test light seen against this matched stabilized image and the positive after-image were identical throughout the course of dark adaptation.

How does it happen that the "dark light" of the positive after-image increases the threshold of the pool? Barlow and Sparrock think that it is because it increases the "noise" against which the signal must be detected. They propose that the "dark light," like the "real light," enters the automatic gain control device through the front. However, Rushton[18] has found evidence for the view that the dark light enters the automatic gain control through the feedback.

These mechanisms of "neural" adaptation and their relation to photochemical events in the retina are only now slowly coming to light. We still know nothing of the actual physiological mechanisms in the retina responsible for these sensitivity changes. The next step in the modeling of the adaptation process will be the quantitative analysis of time characteristics. The photochemical events in the retina have the time characteristics of the kinetics of the visual pigments, and these are much slower than the changes in sensitivity of the automatic gain control of the excitation pool. But there is evidence that, like other automatic gain control devices, sensitivity of the dark-adapted retina is obtained at the expense of speed. As this light-adaptation level increases the loss of sensitivity is accompanied by an increase in speed of the response. This probably lies at the root of a number of other visual phenomena, the decreased latency of vision with increase in intensity as is manifest, say, by the Pulfrich phenomenon[18] and the increase in critical flicker frequency with light intensity (the so-called Ferry-Porter law). Thus, the analog of the excitation pool is important for a host of visual phenomena besides what it tells us about dark and light adaptation.

REFERENCES

1. Stiles, W. S., and Crawford, B. H.: The luminous efficiency of rays entering the eye pupil at different points, Proc. Roy. Soc. (Biol.) 112:428, 1933.
2. Hecht, S., Shlaer, S., and Pirenne, M. H.: Energy, quanta and vision, J. Gen. Physiol. 25:819, 1942.
3. Bouman, M. A., and van der Velden, H. A.: The two-quanta explanation of the dependence of the threshold values and visual acuity on the visual angle and the time of observation, J. Opt. Soc. Amer. 37:908, 1947.
4. McLaughlin, S. C., Jr.: An automatic-recording visual adaptometer, J. Opt. Soc. Amer. 44:312, 1954.
5. Jayle, G. E., and Ourgaud, A. G.: La vision nocturne et ses troubles, Bull. Mem. Soc. Franc. Ophtal. 63:3, 1950.
6. Rushton, W. A. H.: Densitometry of pigments in rods and cones of normal color defective subjects, Invest. Ophthal. 5:233, 1966.
7. Rushton, W. A. H., and Westheimer, G.: The effect upon the rod threshold of bleaching neighbouring rods, J. Physiol. 164:318, 1962.
8. Alpern, M., and Campbell, F. W.: The behaviour of the pupil during dark adaptation, J. Physiol. 165:5-6P, 1962.
9. Dowling, J. E., and Wald, G.: The role of vitamin A acid, Vitamins Hormones (N. Y.) 18:515, 1960.
10. Crawford, B. H.: Visual adaptation in relation to brief conditioning stimuli, Proc. Roy. Soc. (Biol.) 134:283, 1947.
11. Hecht, S.: Intensity discrimination and its relation to the adaptation of the eye, J. Physiol. 86:15, 1936.
12. Wald, G.: Vision: photochemistry. In Glasser, O., editor: Medical physics, Chicago, 1944, Year Book Medical Publishers, Inc.
13. Granit, R., Munsterhjelm, A., and Zewi, M.: The relation between concentration of visual purple and retinal sensitivity to light during dark adaptation, J. Physiol. 96:31, 1939.

14. Rushton, W. A. H.: Rhodopsin measurement and dark adaptation in a subject deficient in cone vision, J. Physiol. **156:**193, 1961.
15. Rushton, W. A. H.: Visual adaptation, The Ferrier Lecture, 1962, Proc. Roy. Soc. (Biol.) **162:** 20, 1965.
16. Fuortes, M. G. F., and Hodgkin, A. L.: Changes in time scale and sensitivity in the ommatidia of Limulus, J. Physiol. **172:**239, 1964.
17. Barlow, H. B., and Sparrock, J. M. B.: The role of after images in dark adaptation, Science **144:**1309, 1964.
18. Alpern, M.: Vision. In Alpern, M., Lawrence, M., and Wolsk, D.: Sensory processes, Belmont, California, 1967, Brooks/Cole Publishing Co.

4 *Clinical aspects of night vision*

ALEX E. KRILL

Most of our visual performance occurs either in daylight or in an artificially lighted environment. Only occasionally is it necessary to perform in absolute or close to absolute darkness for a prolonged period of time. The photographer developing film, the astronomer gazing through a telescope at night, and the pilot flying over the countryside at night all perform in close to absolute darkness. However, the airplane pilot, like the automobile driver, may be subject to frequent changes in illumination, sometimes of a very rapid and extensive nature.

Therefore, it is obvious that in any discussion of everyday visual performance, it is necessary to consider a wide luminance range. Three terms—photopic, scotopic, and mesopic—define visual performance on the basis of luminance range. Photopic vision occurs in daylight. Three foot-lamberts (ft-L) is an average value cited as the lowest luminance for photopic vision. Cones are more sensitive in this range. Scotopic vision occurs in absolute or close to absolute darkness and is rod vision.* A luminance value cited for the upper limit of scotopic vision is 3×10^{-4} ft-L. Mesopic vision occurs in luminances between the lowest value cited for photopic vision and the upper value cited for scotopic luminance. In this range, rod and cone sensitivities are similar. The precise luminance values for when only rods or cones or both function may vary with factors such as area of the retina stimulated, size of the stimulus, and previous light experience.

In general, much of our visual activity under reduced lighting is mesopic. However, visual data may be easier to obtain when mainly rods or cones function in photopic or scotopic environments. Therefore, estimation of mesopic performance requires interpolation, and this may be difficult because the relative contribution of rods and cones in various mesopic environments may be impossible to predict. Usually, though, curves of data (for example, visual acuity and minimum light detection) obtained in complete darkness after previous adaptation to a bright light are of some value in predicting mesopic as well as scotopic performance.

---

*This is true except at the far red end of the visible spectrum, where rods and cones are equally sensitive.[24]

This portion of the chapter will discuss two general areas. First, the most important changes occurring in visual capabilities under reduced illumination will be considered. Second, the various abnormalities of night vision will be discussed.

EFFECT OF REDUCED ILLUMINATION ON VISUAL CAPABILITIES
Visual acuity

In general, visual acuity decreases to a maximum of 20/200 in the fully dark-adapted eye. Mandelbaum and Rowland[1] studied how visual acuity varied with background luminance at the fovea and at 1, 4, 15, and 30 degrees eccentricity to the fovea. The fovea had best acuity until illumination was reduced to about 6 μL. Best acuity was then at the 4-degree position. It is of interest that best acuity is not found in the region of maximum light sensitivity at 15 to 20 degrees eccentricity (where rods are of greatest concentration in the retina). Not only does visual acuity improve with increasing luminance, but it improves even more as the contrast between the target and the background increases.

Color vision

Color vision gradually deteriorates with decrease in luminance. In the fully dark-adapted eye there is little or no hue or saturation discrimination. As pointed out by Alpern (Chapter 3), blue-green light near 510 nm is brightest for the dark-adapted eye and yellow-green light near 560 nm is brightest for the light-adapted eye. Color vision below about 1 ft-L tends to become similar to that of a blue-yellow defective in a 2-degree field in a dark surround.[2] Also short exposure, small size, or eccentric stimulation will deteriorate normal color perception more in dim than in bright illumination. Color vision is more markedly affected in color-defective persons than normal persons by equal changes in illumination. In general, color details are distinguished in mesopic vision mainly according to brightness.

Light detection sensitivity (dark adaptation)

As noted, the most remarkable change that occurs from the light-adapted to the dark-adapted state is the change in light detection sensitivity, which may amount to as much as 100,000 times. This change is described by a dark adaptation curve discussed in great detail in Chapter 3. The measurement of dark adaptation involves the determination of the maximum sensitivity of the eye to a light stimulus at given times in the dark. In general, the greatest sensitivity of the eye is not attained until 25 to 35 minutes in the dark-adapted state, but, as noted by Alpern (Chapter 3), this is dependent on many factors. The ability to dark-adapt decreases with age in the blue-violet region of the spectrum, probably reflecting the increase in yellowness of the lens nucleus that occurs with age.[3]

Optical changes

In general, the dark-adapted eye becomes more myopic than the light-adapted eye.[4] An increase of about 0.50D to 2.00D of myopia has been noted with great variability from individual to individual. There is also a recession of the near point so that an individual has only half his normal accommodative power.[5] This change resembles the recession of the near point that occurs with increasing age, in that the ratio of accommodative convergence to accommodation (AC/A) remains essentially unchanged with this decrease in amplitude of accommodation. The dark-adapted eye has much less depth perception than the light-adapted eye.[6,7] In fact, this ability may decrease to less than one-tenth of what it is in the light-adapted eye.[6] Motion parallax appears to be important in the identification of distances between two objects in reduced illumination. It has been shown that two objects usually appear farther apart in dim than in bright illumination.[8] Therefore, in a fog one may have a false impression of an automobile being farther away than it actually is. White surfaces on a dark background appear smaller and farther away than dark surfaces on a light background.

Diplopia may become more prominent in reduced illumination because of the decrease in fusional stimuli. Phorias may break down to tropias. An intermittent exotropia may become constant. The frequency of these phenomena is unknown and their importance in tasks under reduced illumination is questioned.[9]

Visual field changes

Several changes have been described for scotopic vision.[10] These include:
1. Enlargement of blind spot. A variable enlargement of the normal physiological blind spot occurs.
2. Development of a central blind area, which may measure as much as 2 degrees in the vertical meridian and 2.5 degrees in the horizontal meridian. A small, but definite, scotoma may be detected in the mesopic state.
3. Contraction of the peripheral visual field. The mean radius for the peripheral visual field is about 62 to 64 degrees in the fully dark-adapted eye.
4. Troxler phenomenon intensification. The lower the level of illumination, the faster a target in a peripheral area will disappear if it is held stationary.
5. Autokinetic movement phenomenon. There is a subjective illusion of motion when viewing a single source of light in total darkness for a period of time. This phenomenon is markedly reduced by using two lights and completely abolished by having a subject view three lights.

Glare

Any degree of light falling upon the retina in excess of that which enables one to see clearly may be defined as "glare." Glare will affect most aspects of visual function under reduced illumination.[8-12] Usually glare is measured in one of two ways: (1) by the effect on some parameter under reduced illumination, such as visual acuity or level of dark adaptation, or (2) the time required to reach a previously measured value before a glare source was presented. Glare can be divided into three categories.[13] "Veiling glare" is the type in which light is scattered primarily by the cornea and lens of the eye, producing a uniform veil that is superimposed over the retinal image of a fixation target and that reduces contrast. "Dazzling glare" consists of adventitious light scattered in the light media and not affecting the retinal image. However, marked photophobia resulting may affect vision. Finally, the most disturbing type of glare is scotomatous or "blinding glare," which causes a blind spot in the visual field.

Glare becomes more of a problem in patients with opacities of the ocular media, in patients with defective irides because of surgery or congenital abnormalities (such as aniridia), in certain retinal diseases (such as with cone degenerations), or in general in the aged.

Glare may be particularly reduced by blinking and closing one eye, reducing the recovery time for glare. The recovery time varies from 2 to 6 minutes but may be much greater in the aged.

ABNORMALITIES OF NIGHT VISION

No one test adequately characterizes visual performance under reduced illumination.[8,14] Many investigators, particularly during World War II, searched for such a test.[14] The conclusions in this regard were reviewed by Berry[14] in a publication of the Armed Forces National Research Council Vision Committee. Dark adaptation, the most frequently used test for this purpose, for either light flashes or form could not be used to categorize normal individuals. "Not a single test could be found to categorize personnel for night duty, or for separating normal men into those with functionally inferior night vision and those with functionally adequate night vision."[14] A positive conclusion reached was that "night vision is much too complex to be assayed by any single type of test such as was used."[14]

A battery of tests might suffice for adequately evaluating scotopic and mesopic visual capabilities in normal subjects.[8,9] A possible battery of tests would include a dark-adaptation curve, visual acuity under mesopic and scotopic luminances, and a study of recovery from glare under reduced illumination (these three parameters show little or no correlation with each other in the normal subject). Possibly additional information might be gained from a study of contrast sensitivity (a measure that has limited correlation with visual acuity) under various luminances. If a task relating to motion, such as driving, is evaluated, then dynamic visual acuity probably should also be measured.

In patients with organic disease, there are correlations between all visual measurements under reduced illumination. Almost any test of scotopic function will identify patients with moderate or severe organic nightblindness. However, more subtle abnormalities may be revealed mainly by dark-adaptation studies—in fact, sometimes only by alterations of dark-adaptation rate. In general, then, dark adaptation is the best one test for detecting abnormal scotopic and, to some extent, abnormal mesopic function in patients with disease. In the ensuing discussion of diseases affecting night vision (and one may presume mesopic vision to some degree as well) only the effect of the condition on dark adaptation will be mentioned.

Method

Much of the data in the section on retinal diseases affecting night vision is based on data from my laboratory. We use a modified Goldmann-Weekers adaptometer. As Alpern has indicated, the original commercially available instrument tests only one retinal area, 15 degrees above the fovea, and has only one target size, 11 degrees in diameter. However, it is a very simple matter to construct plates with apertures for testing other target sizes. With our plates we have test targets with diameters of 0.25, 0.5, 1, 2.5, and 5 degrees. In addition, the manufacturers, the Haag-Streit Company, now make a globe with a movable fixation light that can be projected at any point along the horizontal, vertical, or oblique meridians. Plates with colored filters can be used in a second slot behind the globe. For foveal testing, a special fixation device is necessary. We use four light spots equally spaced around the test target (which is usually 0.25 degree for foveal testing). These can be obtained from a battery-powered light source placed in back of a specially constructed plate or by projection from a projector attached to the front of the globe. The subject is maintaining foveal fixation when the four dots are simultaneously visualized. Thus, the new Goldmann-Weekers adaptometer, with proper modifications, is a versatile instrument. There are only a few other commercially available adaptometers. One manufactured in Sweden offers considerable promise.[15]

In our patients, dark-adaptation studies are performed after a careful period of instruction and an initial short trial run. The tested eye is dilated to about 7 to 8 mm with tropicamide 1%. The patient is first placed in complete darkness for 3 minutes and then exposed to a preadapting illumination of 3.13 log

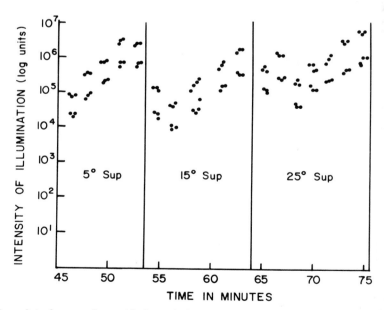

Fig. 4-1. Raw data from patient with hysterical amblyopia after 45 minutes in the dark. The thresholds at the top are when the patient first sees the light (threshold of appearance) and those at the bottom are when the patient states the light has disappeared (threshold of disappearance). These data are typical of a good subject since the thresholds show consistency within one test period. From period to period, however, the thresholds vary but tend to shift upward, a finding typical of hysterical amblyopia. (From Krill, A. E.: Amer. J. Ophthal. **63:**230, 1967.)

mL luminance for 7 minutes. Absolute white-light threshold measurements are started immediately at the completion of preadaptation.

The subject initially fixates on a 2-mm red light of variable brightness, located about 15 degrees above the center (the position of the fixation light in the original instrument) of the test light. In our routine testing, a retinal subtense of 1 degree is always used. The stimulus is presented in the form of light flashes 1 second in duration, the dark interval also being 1 second. The test light is calibrated at a maximum luminance of 9.4 log $\mu\mu$L and at the onset is presented at a luminance of 8.4 log $\mu\mu$L, with the subsequent direction of change dependent on the response of the subject. At each test time four "on" or "ascending" and four "off" or "descending" thresholds are noted (Fig. 4-1).* An "ascending threshold" is the intensity at which the subject first sees the test light as its luminance is increased; a "descending threshold" is the intensity at which the subject ceases to see the test light as its luminance is lowered. Each threshold intensity is mechanically plotted (on a log scale) versus time. The approximate true absolute threshold during a test time is calculated as an average of the four "on" and "off" thresholds obtained at that time. The responses are charted at ½-, 1-, or 2-minute intervals, depending on the time of the test. The subject is notified immediately before the test light is presented and before a rest period.

Each subject is tested in the standard retinal area for a total of 40 minutes, at which time a constant final threshold value is usually obtained. The average test light luminance at the time of threshold stabilization is about 4.4 log $\mu\mu$L. If threshold stabilization is not obtained by 40 minutes, it is continued until thresholds remain stabilized over three successive test periods.

After threshold stabilization the movable fixation light is used and tests are made of 1-degree retinal areas at 5 and 25 degrees eccentricity in the superior meridian. Red and blue light stimuli are then used at these two areas in addition to at the originally tested 15-degree eccentricity area. Additional areas tested depend on the patient and the problem at hand.

Extraretinal causes of abnormal night vision

Clinical vitamin deficiencies. Nightblindness is likely to occur in diseases associated with a significant deficiency of vitamin A[16-24] (a vitamin that plays an important role in the metabolism of rhodopsin). Vitamin A deficiency may occur because of:

1. Deficient intake because of starvation. Alcoholism is a frequent cause of deficient intake in this country. A greater requirement for vitamin A may exist during the last few months of pregnancy[10]; therefore, the complaint of nightblindness is likely to occur during this period, particularly if dietary intake is inadequate to begin with or a superimposed illness occurs.
2. Deficient fat absorption caused by achlorhydria, sprue, celiac disease, chronic gastritis, chronic pancreatitis, chronic gastroenteritis, cystic fibro-

---

*The reliability of a subject is determined by noting the consistency of the thresholds within each test time.

sis, giardiasis, or gastric resection. The record of a patient with celiac disease whom we tested before and after treatment is shown in Fig. 4-2. Gallbladder secretion is essential for fat absorption and therefore obstruction of the common duct may produce a deficiency of vitamin A.

3. Deficient metabolism in the liver resulting particularly from chronic disease of this organ.

4. Massive urinary excretion of vitamin A likely to occur in cancer, severe acute infections with pyrexia such as pneumonia and rheumatic heart disease, or chronic infections such as tuberculosis and chronic nephritis.[25-27]

Deficient vitamin B intake probably also affects night vision, although the relationship is less clear here. It is likely that such deficiencies affect the metabolism of the protein portion, opsin, of the substance rhodopsin.[28] In deficient intake problems or in chronic liver disease, multivitamin deficiencies result, and therefore it is hard to identify which vitamin or vitamins are most important in the cause of visual problems that occur. In patients with deficient dietary intake or liver disease, it is usually just as well to assume that multiple vitamins will be needed, rather than just vitamin A. It has been shown, in fact, that treatment with proteins and vitamin B supplement alone may create additional problems. In the treatment of a starvation disease, kwashiorkor, it is necessary to supplement the treatment of patients with severe protein deficiency with vitamin A.[29] If not, as dietary protein supplement is given, vitamin A requirement increases and the last reserves of this vitamin in the liver eventually are used up.[23,29]

In general, abnormalities of both dark-adaptation rate and threshold are characteristic in patients with multivitamin deficiencies. Classically, it has been

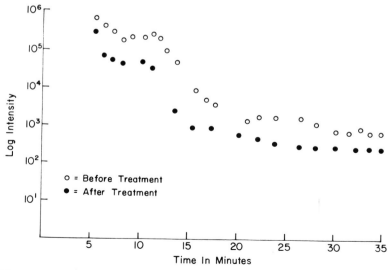

Fig. 4-2. Absolute thresholds from patient with celiac disease before and 6 months after therapy was initiated. Note that curve after treatment is faster and that all thresholds are lower.

claimed that in vitamin A deficiency there is only an elevated final threshold. There are definite examples, though, in which abnormalities of both dark-adaptation rate and threshold are noted (for example, in celiac disease), in spite of what appears to be almost a pure vitamin A deficiency.

Other systemic diseases. Elevated rod absolute thresholds have been cited in patients with hyperthyroidism.[10] In fact, normalization of dark adaptation after treatment of the thyrotoxicosis was noted in a few cases where repeated dark-adaptation studies were done. On the contrary, no conclusive abnormalities are seen in hypothyroidism.

The hemoglobin level may be significant, particularly in patients with nutritional deficiency. Someswara, De, and Subha[30] found a significantly higher incidence of nightblindness where both nutritional deficiency and anemia were found together.

Hypoxia. The retina is markedly susceptible to a decrease in available oxygen (termed "hypoxia") because of its relatively high metabolic rate. It has been demonstrated by several workers[31-35] that hypoxia results in a decrease in white and colored light absolute thresholds. In experiments where hemoglobin oxygen saturations were monitored,[31] it has been shown that hypoxia raises both cone and rod absolute visual thresholds (Fig. 4-3). Rod thresholds are elevated to a greater extent. Peripheral rod thresholds are affected more than central rod thresholds. Only the later portions of rod and cone dark-adaptation curves are affected by hypoxia (Fig. 4-3). The first 4 minutes of either type of curve are unaffected.[31]

An elevation of rod absolute threshold also occurs with increasing altitude.[36] The precise altitude at which deterioration of night vision occurs is dependent on many factors. (In one experiment first effects were detected at about 9,000 feet.) This elevation may be caused by a decrease in available oxygen, but a question that has not been resolved is whether there is an independent effect of barometric pressure on threshold.

In general, it is thought that increasing the oxygen concentration received by an observer who is hypoxic will result in improved visual sensitivity, but this improvement can in no way be extrapolated to the hyperoxic condition. In fact, breathing high concentrations of oxygen under pressure decreases various aspects of visual performance. It is also of interest to note that glucose[36] or rapid breathing (hypercapnia) may protect against the effects of increasing altitude on the dark-adaptation thresholds, whereas insulin enhances this effect.

Refractive errors. Myopic persons, particularly over 15.00D, have higher than normal thresholds even without associated retinal pathology. There is no adequate explanation for these higher thresholds in the myope, but it is not certain that retinal pathology was ruled out in all of these patients.[10]

Glaucoma. Zuege and Drance[37] showed a selective elevation of the final rod threshold at a retinal eccentricity of 15 degrees in early open-angle glaucoma. This abnormality was best shown by comparing a ratio of the absolute threshold at 15 degrees to that at 30 degrees in glaucoma and normal patients of the same age. This abnormality was demonstrated in patients with elevated ocular tension, even before visual field changes were noted.

Occasionally, a patient with untreated glaucoma will complain of some degree of nightblindness and show an improvement in dark adaptation after treatment.

Patients on miotics experience a loss in visual sensitivity roughly proportional to the reduction in area of pupillary size caused by the drug.[38,39]

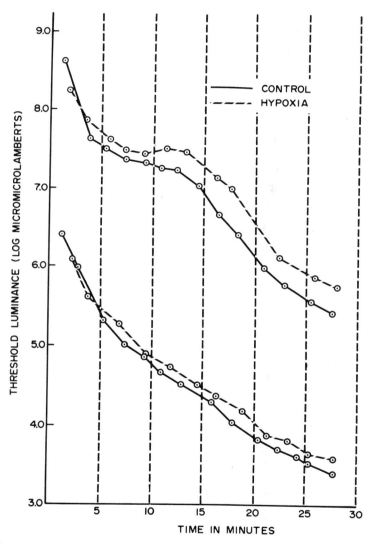

Fig. 4-3. Effect of hypoxia on dark adaptation. The upper two dark-adaptation curves were obtained with a 1-degree circular yellow target at an eccentricity of 5 degrees in the nasal field on the horizontal meridian. The subject's eye was preadapted with blue light having a luminance of 1,000 mL. The lower two dark-adaptation curves were recorded with a 1-degree circular blue target at the same 5-degree eccentricity. The subject's eye was preadapted with red light having a luminance of 1,000 mL. Note how curves are elevated by hypoxia. (From Ernest, J. T., and Krill, A. E.: Invest. Ophthal. **10:**323, 1971.)

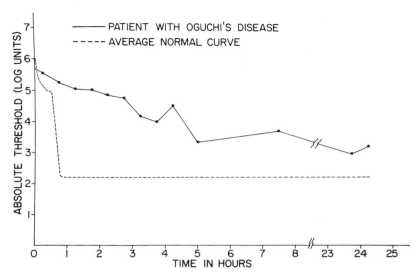

Fig. 4-4. Dark-adaptation curve from patient with Oguchi's disease. Patient took about 4 or 5 hours to reach a final threshold. Final threshold is slightly elevated.

RETINAL CAUSES OF ABNORMAL DARK ADAPTATION
Abnormalities of dark-adaptation time

Oguchi's disease. Oguchi's disease is a form of congenital stationary night-blindness associated with a peculiar yellowish or grayish discoloration of the fundus. Prolonged dark adaptation usually leads to a disappearance of the abnormal fundus coloration (known as Mizuo's phenomenon) and marked improvement or normalization of subjective dark adaptation.[40,41]

Patients with Oguchi's disease have been divided into two major types.[40] Type 1 patients are characterized by the occurrence of rod dark adaptation after a sufficient period of time in the dark. The final rod threshold may be normal or elevated. (Fig. 4-4 shows a patient who took 4 or 5 hours to show a rod cone break. Note also that the final threshold is slightly elevated.) Also, after sufficient time in the dark, the abnormal fundus coloration disappears in type 1 patients. Patients in a second group, type 2, show no rod dark adaptation. These patients have less striking abnormal fundus coloration than those classified as type 1. Some of these patients, type 2A, show Mizuo's phenomenon, whereas others, type 2B, do not.

The time for complete secondary dark adaptation to occur in type 1 patients varies from case to case and also with the degree of preadaptation. Generally, most cases take 2 to 4 hours, but as long as 24 hours has been reported. The time for complete disappearance of the abnormal coloration is not related to the time for complete secondary dark adaptation.

Flecked retina syndrome. Three conditions characterized by a limited or widespread distribution of deep yellowish or white lesions of various sizes and configuration without vascular and optic nerve abnormalities or pigment migra-

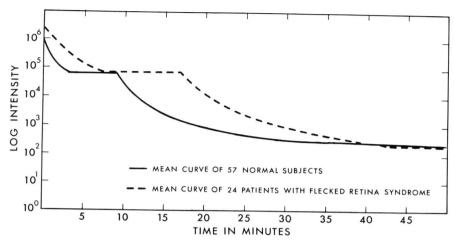

Fig. 4-5. Mean dark-adaptation curves from fifty-seven normal persons and twenty-four patients with the "flecked retina syndrome." Note the delay in reaching the final cone and rod thresholds and in the rod-cone break in the patient curve. The values of the final thresholds are about the same in the two groups. (From Krill, A. E., and Klien, B. A.: Arch. Ophthal. [Chicago] 74:496, 1965.)

tion have in common certain features, designated the flecked retina syndrome.[42] The three conditions are drusen, fundus albipunctatus, and fundus flavimaculatus. Each has distinct ophthalmoscopic, fluorescein, and probably pathological characteristics outlined in detail elsewhere.[43,44]

The common features include a high incidence of macular disease, normal peripheral visual fields, a usual abnormal electro-oculogram, and characteristic dark-adaptation time abnormalities. In general, dark-adaptation cone and rod thresholds are normal, but the time when each occurs as well as the rod cone break time is slower than normal (Fig. 4-5). The b-wave of the electroretinogram, which is usually of normal amplitude, takes longer than normal to reach a maximum amplitude in the dark-adapted eye.[42] Occasionally, the time of dark adaptation is so delayed that the patient will complain of "difficulty in adjusting to the dark," but most patients have no "night visual complaints."

Fleck retina of Kandori. The fleck retina of Kandori is a stationary, probably congenital, condition seen up to date only in Japan and characterized by large, discrete, irregularly shaped deposits in the midperipheral fundus.[45] There is a slower than normal dark-adaptation curve, with normal final thresholds usually evident by 40 minutes after the start of testing. A slower than normal time to reach a maximum scotopic b-wave has also been noted.

In contrast to drusen, fundus albipunctatus, and fundus flavimaculatus, visual acuity is always normal in the fleck retina.

Stationary abnormalities of final threshold

Congenital stationary nightblindness without fundus changes. Congenital stationary nightblindness with no fundus changes can be divided into three types

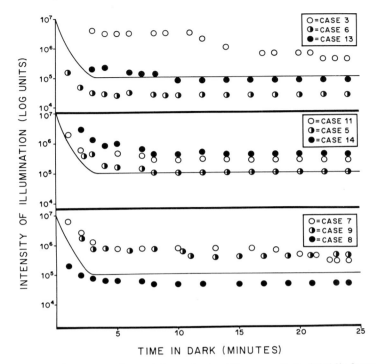

Fig. 4-6. Dark-adaptation curves from eight patients with congenital nightblindness. All curves are monofunctional, showing only cone curves. Note that several of the curves are slower than normal in reaching a final cone threshold and that some of the cone thresholds are elevated. (From Krill, A. E., and Martin, D.: Invest. Ophthal. **10:**625, 1971.)

on the basis of hereditary pattern.[46,47] In all three inherited types, though, there is a marked inability to see at night because of the complete absence of rod adaptation in affected individuals (Fig. 4-6).

Vision is always normal in the dominant form but always abnormal in the X-linked recessive form. Vision may be normal or abnormal in the autosomal recessive type. Acuity may be as poor as 20/200 but is more likely, in patients with abnormal vision, to range between 20/40 to 20/100. Myopia is universal in the X-linked recessive type and frequent in the autosomal recessive form with abnormal vision.

Mild to moderate photopic abnormalities are common in all three hereditary types of congenital nightblindness.[46] In fact, the characteristic monophasic cone dark-adaptation curve is frequently slow and elevated compared to normal controls (Fig. 4-6).

Congenital stationary nightblindness with fundus changes

Fundus albipunctatus. An occasional patient with fundus albipunctatus will show no secondary or rod adaptation. Most patients will show a delayed dark adaptation, as indicated in the previous discussion.

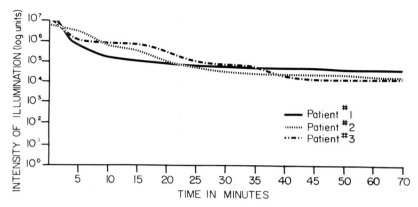

Fig. 4-7. Dark-adaptation curves from three patients with retinitis pigmentosa. Note that both rod and cone segments are elevated.

Oguchi's disease. As indicated, patients with type 2A Oguchi's disease show no secondary or rod dark adaptation.

Hereditary vitreoretinal degeneration and nightblindness.[48] A pedigree was described in which a typical vitreoretinal degeneration of autosomal recessive inheritance was associated with a stationary form of congenital nightblindness. The dark-adaptation and electroretinographic findings were typical of stationary nightblindness.

Progressive abnormalities of dark-adaptation thresholds. Diffuse chorioretinal degeneration—including retinitis pigmentosa, the choroidal atrophies, such as gyrate atrophy, and choroideremia—and some of the vitreoretinal degenerations are all characterized by early and diffuse involvement of the receptors. Therefore, afflicted patients complain of nightblindness as an early symptom. Abnormal dark-adaptation curves are characteristic even in early stages of the disease. Frequently the rods are involved earlier and to a greater exent than the cones, so that there is a greater elevation of the rod portion of the dark-adaptation curve. Eventually, though, cone thresholds are usually also considerably elevated (Fig. 4-7).

An interesting finding that has been demonstrated in retinitis pigmentosa, and which depicts the greater involvement of the rods as compared to the cones, is the so-called "inverted profile" (Fig. 4-8).[49,51] In the normal subject the thresholds are usually slightly higher at 5 degrees than at 10 or 25 degrees retinal eccentricity. However, in the patient with retinitis pigmentosa the threshold at 5 degrees is almost always lower than at the more peripheral areas, reflecting the greater involvement of rods, which are more concentrated in the peripheral areas tested.

There is sometimes a problem as to whether eyeground changes represent scarring from a previous inflammatory process or a progressive retinal degeneration. An electroretinogram is markedly abnormal and frequently extinguished in the latter, but only mildly abnormal or normal after a chorioretinitis; but this test is not always available. Several dark-adaptation findings may aid in

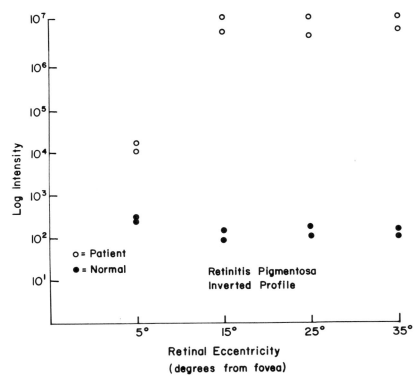

Fig. 4-8. Dark-adaptation data from two patients with retinitis pigmentosa and two normal persons at 5, 15, 25, and 35 degrees retinal eccentricities. Note that in the nomal subjects thresholds are slightly higher at 5 degrees, whereas in patients with retinitis pigmentosa thresholds are lowest at this point. This characteristic greater involvement of areas away from the macula is related to a more pronounced effect of the disease on rods than on cones and is known as the "inverted profile."

distinguishing the two conditions. The finding of an inverted retinal profile, described previously, favors a retinal degeneration. Severe elevation of both rod and cone thresholds is more characteristic of retinitis pigmentosa (Fig. 4-7). Finally, successive dark-adaptation determinations over a period of time (Fig. 4-9) indicates a progressive disorder (sometimes where distinct changes are not evident on less sensitive visual field testing).

Abeta-lipoproteinemia is associated with a retinal degeneration and typical functional changes such as severe nightblindness. It has recently been shown that the retinal changes may be reversible. Carr[52] reported restoration of dark adaptation in two affected patients following administration of doses of 200,000 units of vitamin A and a continued maintenance of the serum vitamin A levels. It appears that the ability to dark-adapt closely parallels the serum vitamin A level in this condition.

Myotonic dystrophy is characterized by abnormalities of retinal function, in spite of frequently normal appearing eyegrounds.[53] Burian and Burns[53] have

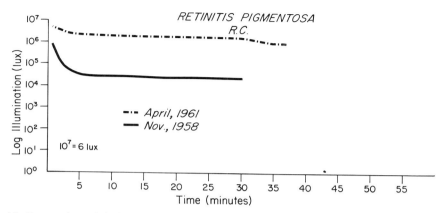

Fig. 4-9. Progression of dark-adaptation abnormality in patient with retinitis pigmentosa over a period of almost 3 years.

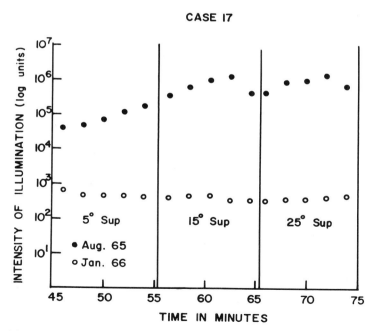

Fig. 4-10. Initial and followup average threshold data after 45 minutes in the dark for a patient with hysterical amblyopia. Note that thresholds on the first test are elevated and also tend to shift upward ("exhaustion phenomenon"). On the second test thresholds were within normal limits and no longer showed fluctuation. At this time the patient's psychological status was also thought to be improved. (From Krill, A. E.: Amer. J. Ophthal. **63:**230, 1967.)

shown elevated final rod thresholds, particularly with blue targets, in this condition. It is not certain as yet, though, whether this is a progressive abnormality or not. It is obvious that the absence or presence of retinal involvement is not always apparent from the appearance of the eyegrounds. Dark-adaptation studies, as well as tests such as the electroretinogram and electro-oculogram, may be helpful in evaluating the presence and the type of retinal abnormality in various diseases.

Conversion reaction affecting vision ("hysterical amblyopia")

Two dark-adaptation abnormalities may be found in patients with hysterical amblyopia.[54,55] Elevated rod thresholds were found in thirty-six of fifty-six patients with this diagnosis that were tested. Thirty of the thirty-six showed another interesting phenomenon called the "exhaustion phenomenon" (Figs. 4-1 and 4-10).[55] Seven without elevated final thresholds also showed this finding. This exhaustion phenomenon comprises a consistent upper shift in threshold of at least 0.5 log units after prolonged testing. This finding is not seen in normal persons or in patients with organic disease (unless a superimposed conversion reaction is present). Repeated dark-adaptation studies in such patients may correlate with the psychological status of the individual (Fig. 4-10). Elevated absolute thresholds, not organic in origin, have also been found in psychotic persons.[56]

Malingering, false cues

It is possible for a patient to choose and maintain a given test light level above his absolute visual threshold if he can depend on clues other than the test light. The clues used may be such factors as the time between test light exposures, the sound of a test light shutter, inadvertent signals from the examiner, or the like. It is possible to exclude mechanical or procedural techniques that might be used by a patient to give test results that are not valid. However, one worker recommends the use of a specific technique called the double staircase method to prevent falsely abnormal results.[57]

Toxic retinopathy

In toxic retinopathies caused by a number of agents, there may be severe retinal involvement, as evidenced by all tests of retinal function, including dark adaptation. Two examples of such drugs include quinine[58] and thioridazine.[59] Transient toxic retinopathy of a mild degree may be found in acute or subacute intoxication with ethyl alcohol.[60] In fact, slow dark adaptation with some elevation of final thresholds may be one of the major functional abnormalities in this condition.

Chloroquine retinopathy. On the other hand, a striking exception is found in chloroquine retinopathy. An unusual finding in this condition is the presence of normal or close to normal final or rod adaptation in all areas of the retina, even in advanced stages of the disease, with an extinguished electroretinogram.[61] However, cone function, as measured by initial dark adaptation or by red-light thresholds, is usually abnormal, even in early stages of chloroquine retinopathy.[62]

In fact, elevated red-light absolute thresholds may be the most sensitive criterion of early chloroquine retinopathy in most patients.[62] However, some patients have macular sparing and therefore red-light thresholds may be normal.[61]

Contrary to what is found on subjective dark adaptation, no such distinction between the cone and rod portions of the electroretinogram is evident in advanced cases. Indeed, no responses are observed, regardless of the conditions of testing. The explanation for its discrepancy between what is found on the electroretinogram and on subjective dark adaptation in advanced chloroquine retinopathy is not clear.[61]

Since the eyegrounds of advanced chloroquine retinopathy may be similar to those seen in retinitis pigmentosa, it is important to know that dark-adaptation profiles easily distinguish the two conditions. As indicated previously, most patients with even early retinitis pigmentosa have markedly abnormal final thresholds. An occasional patient, particularly with an autosomal dominant or sector form of retinitis pigmentosa, will show close to normal thresholds in some retinal areas. However, in contrast to chloroquine reinopathy, when testing is done in several areas in the same quadrant (or in different quadrants with sector retinitis pigmentosa), markedly elevated final thresholds are always seen in some areas (Fig. 4-11).

We have tested some patients with primary cone degenerations who eventually had a severe abnormality of the scotopic electroretinogram but who retained a normal or only slightly abnormal dark adaptation in all areas tested.[63] The selective involvement of the portion of the electroretinogram related to cone function, the severe color vision abnormality, and the early age of onset

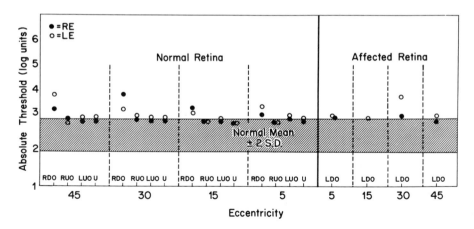

Fig. 4-11. Absolute threshold values from patient with sector retinitis pigmentosa plotted with data from normal control population (mean plus or minus 2 standard deviations). Note that although thresholds are often normal, with scanning some elevated thresholds are always detected. The symbols used to designate meridians are *R* for right, *L* for left, *O* for oblique, *D* for inferior, and *U* for superior. The position on a meridian (eccentricity) is shown along the X axis in degrees. (From Krill, A. E., Archer, D., and Martin, D.: Amer. J. Ophthal. **69**:977, 1970.)

are among some of the findings distinguishing the cone degenerations from chloroquine retinopathy.[63]

REFERENCES

1. Mandelbaum, J., and Rowland, L. S.: Central and paracentral visual acuity at different levels of illumination, Randolph Field, Texas, U. S. Air Force School of Aviation, Medicine, June, 1944, Project No. 220, Report No. 1.
2. Brown, W. R. J.: The influence of luminance level on visual sensitivity to color differences, J. Opt. Soc. Amer. **41**:684, 1951.
3. Gunkel, R. D., and Gouras, P.: Changes in scotopic visibility thresholds with age, Arch. Ophthal. (Chicago) **69**:4, 1963.
4. Mellerio, J.: Ocular refraction at low illumination, Vision Res. **6**:217, 1966.
5. Alpern, M., and Larson, B. F.: Vergence and accommodation, IV. Effect of luminance quantity on the AC/A, Amer. J. Ophthal. **49**:1140, 1960.
6. Invanoff, A.: Night binocular convergence and night myopia, J. Opt. Soc. Amer. **45**:769, 1955.
7. Lit, A.: Depth-discrimination thresholds as a function of binocular differences of retinal illuminance at scotopic and photopic levels, J. Opt. Soc. Amer. **49**:746, 1959.
8. Schmidt, I.: Are meaningful night vision tests for drivers feasible? Amer. J. Optom. **38**:295, 1961.
9. Keeney, A. H.: Ophthalmic pathology in driver limitation, Trans. Amer. Acad. Ophthal. Otolaryng. **72**:737, 1968.
10. Jayle, G. E., and others: Night vision, Springfield, Ill., 1959, Charles C Thomas, Publisher.
11. Vos, J. J.: Physiologic optical aspects of participation in traffic. In Henkes, H. E., editor: Perspectives of ophthalmology, Amsterdam, 1968, Excerpta Medica Foundation.
12. Fry, G. A., and Alpern, M.: The effect of a peripheral glare source upon the apparent brightness of an object, J. Opt. Soc. Amer. **43**:189, 1953.
13. Bell, L. M., Troland, L. T., and Verhoeff, F. H.: Report of the Subcommittee on Glare, Trans. Illum. Eng. Soc. **17**:743, 1922.
14. Berry, W.: Review of war-time studies of dark adaptation, night vision tests, and related topics, Ann Arbor Mich., 1949, Armed Forces NRC Vision Committee.
15. Norden, A., and Stigmar, G.: Measurement of dark-adaptation in vitamin A deficiency by a new quantitative technique, Acta Ophthal. **47**:81, 1969.
16. Adams, D. F., Johnstone, J. M., and Hunter, R. F.: Vitamin A deficiency following total gastrectomy, Lancet **1**:415, 1960.
17. Booker, L. E., Callison, E. C., and Hewston, E. M.: An experimental determination of the minimum vitamin A requirements of normal adults, J. Nutr. **17**:317, 1939.
18. Brenner, S., and Roberts, L.: Effects of vitamin A deletion in young adults, Arch. Intern. Med. **71**:474, 1943.
19. Graham, C. H.: Vision and visual perception, New York, 1965, John Wiley & Sons, Inc.
20. Hecht, S., and Mandelbaum, J.: The relation between vitamin A and dark adaptation, J.A.M.A. **112**:910, 1939.
21. Patek, A. J., and Haig, C.: The occurrence of abnormal dark adaptation and its relation to vitamin A metabolism in patients with cirrhosis of the liver, J. Clin. Invest. **18**:609, 1939.
22. Petersen, R. A., Petersen, V. S., and Robb, R. M.: Vitamin A deficiency with xerophthalmia and nightblindness in cystic fibrosis, Amer. J. Dis. Child. **116**:662, 1968.
23. Roels, O. A.: Vitamin A physiology, J.A.M.A. **214**:1097, 1970.
24. Wald, G., Jeghers, J., and Armino, J.: An experiment in human dietary nightblindness, Amer. J. Physiol. **123**:732, 1938.
25. McLaren, D. S.: Malnutrition in the eye, New York, 1963, Academic Press, Inc., pp. 166-207.
26. Moore, T.: Vitamin A, London, 1957, Elsevier Publishing Co., pp. 357-364, 418-441.
27. Rodger, F. C., and Sinclair, H. M.: Metabolic and nutritional eye diseases, Springfield, Ill., 1969, Charles C Thomas, Publisher.
28. Dowling, J. E., and Wald, G.: Nightblindness, Proc. Nat. Acad. Sci. **44**:648, 1958.
29. Arroyave, G., Wilson, J., and Mendez, M.: Alterations in serum concentrations of vitamin A associated with hypoproteinemia of severe protein malnutrition, J. Pediat. **62**:920, 1963.

30. Someswara, R. K., De, N. K., and Subha, R. P.: Relationship between anemia and night-blindness, Indian J. Med. Res. **41:**349, 1953.

31. Ernest, J. T., and Krill, A. E.: The effect of hypoxia on visual function, Invest. Ophthal. **10:**323, 1971.

32. McDonald, D. R., and Adler, F.: Effects of anoxia on the dark adaptation of the normal and of the vitamin A deficient subject, Arch. Ophthal. (Chicago) **22:**980, 1939.

33. McFarland, R. A., and Evans, J. N.: Alterations in dark-adaptation under reduced oxygen tensions, Amer. J. Physiol. **127:**37, 1939.

34. McFarland, R. A., Halperin, M. H., and Niven, J. I.: Visual thresholds as an index of physiological imbalance during anoxia, Amer. J. Physiol. **142:**328, 1944.

35. Sheard, C.: Effect of anoxia: oxygen and increased intrapulmonary pressure on dark adaptation, Mayo Clin. Proc. **20:**230, 1945.

36. McFarland, R. A., and Forbes, W. H.: Effects of variations in the concentration of oxygen and of glucose on dark adaptation, J. Gen. Physiol. **24:**69, 1940.

37. Zuege, P., and Drance, S. M.: Studies of dark adaptation of discrete paracentral retinal areas in glaucomatous subjects, Amer. J. Ophthal. **98:**54, 1969.

38. Lindstrom, E. E., Tredici, T. J., and Martin, B. G.: Effects of topical ophthalmic 2% pilocarpine on visual performance of normal subjects, Aerospace Med. **39:**1236, 1968.

39. Stewart, W. C., Madill, H. D., and Dyer, A. M.: Night vision in the miotic eye, Canad. Med. Ass. J. **99:**1145, 1968.

40. François, J.: La maladie d'Oguchie, Bull. Soc. Belg. Ophtal. **110:**170, 1955.

41. Carr, R. E., and Gouras, P.: Oguchi's disease, Arch. Ophthal. (Chicago) **73:**646, 1965.

42. Krill, A. E., and Klien, B. A.: Flecked retina syndrome, Arch. Ophthal. (Chicago) **74:**496, 1965.

43. Klien, B. A., and Krill, A. E.: Fundus flavimaculatus: clinical, functional and histopathologic observations, Amer. J. Ophthal. **64:**3, 1967.

44. Farkas, T. G., and others: Familial and secondary drusen: histologic and functional correlations, Trans. Amer. Acad. Ophthal. Otolaryng. **75:**333, 1971.

45. Kandori, F., and others: Studies on fleck retina, Amer. J. Ophthal. **73:**673, 1972.

46. Krill, A. E., and Martin, D.: Photopic abnormalities in congenital stationary nightblindness, Invest. Ophthal. **10:**625, 1971.

47. Franceschetti, A., François, J., and Babel, J.: Les hérédodegénérescences chorio-retiniennes, Paris, 1963, Masson et Cie.

48. Feiler-Ofry, V., and others: Hereditary vitreoretinal degeneration and nightblindness, Amer. J. Ophthal. **67:**553, 1969.

49. Sloan, L. L.: Light sense in pigmentary degeneration of the retina, Arch. Ophthal. (Chicago) **28:**613, 1942.

50. Sloan, L. L.: Rate of dark adaptation and regional threshold gradient of the dark-adapted eye; physiologic and clinical studies, Amer. J. Ophthal. **30:**705, 1947.

51. Zeavin, B. H., and Wald, G.: Rod and cone vision in retinitis pigmentosa, Amer. J. Ophthal. **42:**253, 1956.

52. Carr, R. E.: Vitamin A therapy may reverse degenerative retinal syndrome, Clin. Trends **8:**8, 1970.

53. Burian, H. M., and Burns, C. A.: Electroretinography and dark adaptation in myotonic dystrophy, Amer. J. Ophthal. **61:**1044, 1966.

54. Granger, G. W.: Dark adaptation in anxiety states and hysterics, Brit. J. Physiol. Opt. **13:**235, 1956.

55. Krill, A. E.: Retinal function studies in hysterical amblyopia: a unique abnormality of dark adaptation, Amer. J. Ophthal. **63:**230, 1967.

56. Wolin, L. R., and others: Objective measurement of light thresholds of neuropsychiatric patients, Int. J. Neuropsychiat. **1:**504, 1965.

57. Ernest, J. T.: Night vision testing, Milit. Med. **136:**381, 1971.

58. François, J., Verriest, G., and DeRouck, A.: Etude des fonctions visuelles dans deux cas d' intoxication par la quinine, Ophthalmologica **153:**324, 1967.

59. Connell, M. M., Poley, B. J., and McFarlane, J. R.: Chorioretinopathy associated with thioridazine therapy, Arch. Ophthal. (Chicago) **71:**816, 1964.

60. Verriest, G., and Laplasse, D.: New data concerning the influence of ethyl alcohol on human visual thresholds, Exp. Eye Res. **4:**95, 1965.
61. Krill, A. E., Potts, A. M., and Johanson, C. E.: Chloroquine retinopathy: investigation of a discrepancy between dark adaptation and the electroretinogram in advanced stages, Amer. J. Ophthal. **71:**530, 1971.
62. Carr, R. E., Gouras, P., and Gunkel, R. D.: Chloroquine retinopathy; early detection by retinal threshold test, Arch. Ophthal. (Chicago) **75:**171, 1966.
63. Krill, A. E., and Deutman, A. F.: Dominant macular degenerations: the cone dystrophies, Amer. J. Ophthal. **73:**352, 1972.

PART III Color vision

CHAPTER 5 *Color vision of normal observers*

JOEL POKORNY
VIVIANNE C. SMITH

DEFINING COLOR

The word "color" is used to define one of the qualities of visual sensation. Sensations by their nature are impossible to describe but may be categorized. It is important to note that the color qualities of an object are not physical properties of that object. When we talk of the green grass or the red flowers, we are identifying the color qualities associated with the external physical stimuli. A definition of color is thus by specification of the physical conditions correlated with specific color reports for a given observer.

There are two basic classes of data concerning chromatic vision and the mechanisms subserving it:

1. Psychological concepts of color refer to color percepts and the methods by which the individual may describe his color perceptions. The major ways in which color percepts may vary include hue, saturation, and brightness. Hue is the attribute of color that may be described by the words red, yellow, green, blue, purple, and the like. Saturation refers to the attribute of color that may be distinguished along a continuum such as red . . . pink . . . white. The less saturated a color, the closer it is to white. The brightness of a self-luminous object refers to its apparent intensity on a continuum ranging from very dim to dazzling.[1]
2. Psychophysical concepts of color are determined by classes of experiments in which the observer reports whether a stimulus was present or absent (thresholds) or the observer makes judgments of similarity and difference between two adjacent stimulus fields (matching and discrimination). Topics include spectral sensitivity, color mixture, wavelength discrimination, and saturation discrimination. Each of these in turn is described by a specific experimental paradigm and will be discussed in the body of the chapter.

PRODUCTION OF CHROMATIC STIMULI

Light is defined as the portion of the electromagnetic spectrum that serves as an adequate stimulus for vision (400 to 700 nm). Chromatic stimuli are pro-

*Preparation of this chapter was supported in part by U. S. Public Health Service, National Institutes of Health, NEI grants EY-00277 and EY-00523.

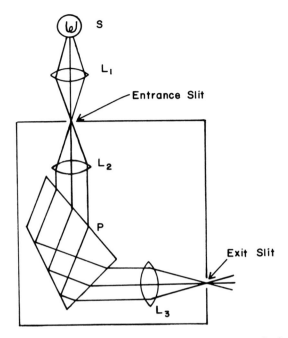

Fig. 5-1. Schematic diagram of a monochromator employing a constant deviation (Pellica-Broca) prism. An image of the source (*S*) is produced on the entrance slit of the monochromator by lens L_1. Light is then collimated by lens L_2 and passes to the prism (*P*). Light exiting from the prism at a 90-degree angle is collected by lens L_3 and imaged on the exit slit. The wavelength composition of the exiting light depends on the angle of rotation of the prism.

duced when various portions of this section of the electromagnetic spectrum are isolated. We may differentiate between methods using optical principles (such as dispersion, diffraction, interference, or absorption) to isolate specific portions of the electromagnetic spectrum from a continuous (white) light source and methods using light sources (such as gas discharge lamps or lasers) whose output is concentrated in specific portions of the spectrum or in a series of spectral lines.

Monochromator

An instrument that allows selection of narrow portions of the spectrum is called a monochromator. By turning the wavelength knob of a monochromator, each wavelength of the incident light is sequentially brought to the same output position. Monochromators can be made using prisms in which the entering light is separated into its spectrum by dispersion (Fig. 5-1). The operator has control of both the mean wavelength (by varying the angle of rotation of the prism) and the width of the wavelength band (by varying the width of the entrance and exit slits). An adequate description of a chromatic stimulus includes: (1) the wavelength of maximum output and (2) the half width (also called half-height band width or band pass)[2] (Fig. 5-2). The half width is obtained by finding the wavelength difference between the two wavelengths in the band hav-

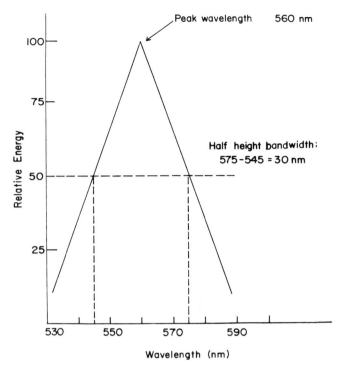

Fig. 5-2. Sample calculation of half-height band width. The two wavelengths in the band that have half the maximum output are found and the difference between these is the half-height band width.

ing half the maximum output. In Fig. 5-2, the wavelength maximum is 560 nm and the half width is 30 nm (575 nm − 545 nm). Other types of monochromators make use of interference wedges or diffraction gratings to separate the entering white light. The diffraction grating monochromator has the advantage that the half width does not change with wavelength.

Selective filters

Color filters can also be used to transmit a selected portion of the spectrum. Several types are presently available, each having virtues in terms of performance and/or costs.

Gelatin and colored glass filters obtain selectivity by absorption. Typically, these filters have broad transmission characteristics (with half widths of 50 to 100 nm). If the filter transmits only at one end of the spectrum, it is known as a cut-off filter. Transmission values near 100% are obtainable for cut-off filters passing long wavelengths. Advantages of such filters include high efficiency, ready availability, and low cost.

Interference filters transmit only a very narrow band of wavelengths. The remainder of the light is reflected off the filter. Frequently such filters have multiple transmission peaks (Fig. 5-3), and blocking filters (glass or gelatin) are

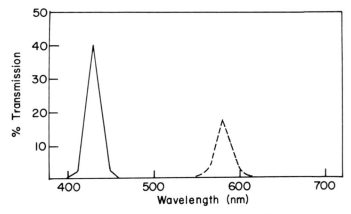

Fig. 5-3. Interference filter with primary transmission peak at 430 nm and a secondary transmission peak at 580 nm. The higher peak has been blocked with a gelatin filter, yielding a single peak transmission characteristic.

required to yield a single peak transmisison characteristic. Interference filters can be made with a half width as narrow as 0.10 nm. Filters used for visual research typically have half widths ranging from 1 to 20 nm. Interference filter specifications are based upon test conditions in which collimated light passes to the filter at a right angle to the surface of the filter. If the filter is rotated, maximal transmission shifts to shorter wavelengths. Similarly, when an interference filter is placed in a converging or diverging beam of light, the band pass widens and the peak transmission shifts to shorter wavelengths.

Colored papers

A third method of obtaining spectrally selected stimuli from white light uses colored papers. Colored papers form the basis of many tests of color blindness and are among the most widely used of all colored stimuli. Papers can rarely be obtained whose spectral reflectance lies within a narrow band of wavelengths. There are several precautions that should be observed when using colored papers. The color appearance will change as illumination is changed. The color depends on both the reflective characteristics of the paper and the energy distribution of the illumination. Adequate specification of both the reflectance of the paper and the illumination is thus necessary. The papers manufactured by the Munsell Company are of particular value since their spectral characteristics are well specified and manufacturing control is excellent. Disadvantages of colored papers are: (1) the ease with which their appearance may be changed by fingerprints, dust, and other superficial dirt; (2) the limited range of reflective values; and (3) the tendency of dyes to fade with time and exposure to light.

Chromatic light sources

Another basic way of obtaining color stimuli is by the use of a source whose output may be concentrated in one or more spectral lines. For example, the

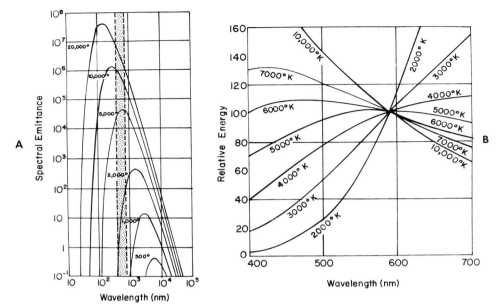

Fig. 5-4. A, Spectral energy distribution of a blackbody as a function of temperature. The band indicates the range of visible radiation. **B,** Relative energy in the visible region of the spectrum as a function of color temperature. The heights of the curves have been adjusted so that the energy at 590 nm is equal to 100.

cadmium-mercury gas lamp has principal lines with wavelengths at 405, 408, 436, 468, 480, 492, 509, 546, 578, and 635 nm. Single lines can be isolated with appropriate blocking filters. Such lamps thus provide highly monochromatic stimuli for visual research. Further, the lamps have an important use in the calibration of monochromators.

Another class of light source providing monochromatic light is the laser, which can produce extremely high energy levels of light. The term "laser" is an acronym for *light amplification by stimulated emission of radiation*. Lasers have one or more highly monochromatic emission wavelengths. Recently developed dye lasers may be tuned (that is, output wavelength varied) over a wide spectral region.

Color temperature

There are many physical stimuli that are correlated with the sensation white, some involving the mixture of a few as two wavelengths. Common white stimuli such as sunlight or light from a tungsten lamp have continuous spectra; some energy is present at all visible wavelengths. The preferred method of specifying a white for a continuous light source is by means of color temperature.

As a body is heated (for example, the voltage on a tungsten lamp is increased), the radiant energy emitted by the body extends over an increasingly wide band of wavelengths. At low temperatures the rate of radiation is low and the radiation is chiefly of relatively long wavelength. At 800° K a body emits enough radiant energy to be self-luminous and appears "red-hot." By far the majority of energy emitted, however, is still in the infrared region of the spectrum. At 3,000° K there is enough radiant energy in the shorter wavelengths so that the body appears "white-hot."

The manner of specification of the spectral output of emissive sources is in

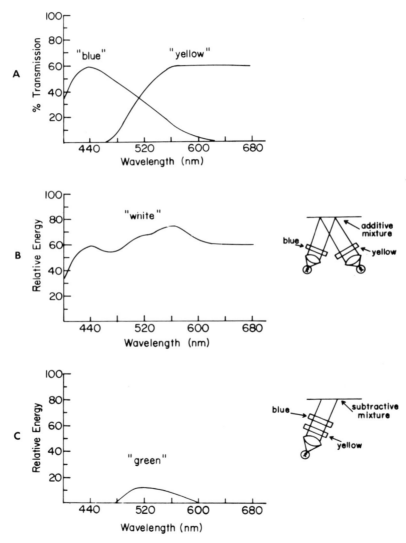

Fig. 5-5. Additive and subtractive mixtures using filters. **A,** Spectral transmission characteristics for a blue (Kodak Wratten No. 9) filter and a yellow (Kodak Wratten No. 38A with 0.2 ND) filter. **B,** Additive mixture of light through both filters (equal energy source). **C,** Subtractive mixture with light transmitted successively through the two filters.

terms of temperature, but since different sources have different outputs when heated to the same temperature, all sources are referred to a theoretical standard called a "blackbody" (or ideal radiator). A blackbody is a theoretical surface that absorbs all the energy impinging on it. It also emits all this energy and has a characteristic spectral output as a function of temperature (Fig. 5-4). Available sources, such as tungsten or carbon, have different spectral outputs at a given temperature, but it is possible to specify them in terms of the temperature of a blackbody with equivalent spectral response. The color temperature of a specimen lamp is the operating temperature of an ideal radiator whose spectral output matches that of the specimen lamp. The National Bureau of Standards has defined the national standard of light to be a blackbody radiator operated at the temperature of solidification of platinum (2,042° K).

The concept of color temperature may also be extended to specification of the appearance of noncontinuous lamps. It is possible, for example, to specify various fluorescent lamps by stating the color temperature correlated with their spectral appearance. When color temperature is applied to discontinuous sources, it is called the "correlated color temperature."

Additive and subtractive mixtures

There is an important physical difference between mixing lights and mixing pigments. When two or more colored lights are superimposed, an additive mixture results. For example, we may superimpose the outputs of two projectors, each containing a spectral filter. If one filter transmits principally in the blue and the other in the yellow, the resulting mixture will contain all the wavelength components of both filters. The hue reported by an observer would probably be white or gray. When light is directed on a mixture of pigments or through a series of filters, a subtractive mixture results. For example, the blue and yellow filters may be placed sequentially in the light path of one projector or blue and yellow pigments mixed. The resultant mixture contains only the wavelengths common to both filters or pigments. In this case, the correlated hue will probably be a dark green. Fig. 5-5 shows the results of additive and subtractive mixtures using two filters.

While most painting thus involves subtractive mixture, the painters of the pointillist school of art achieved the effect of additive mixture by placing small dots of colors adjacent to each other.[3] Light is reflected from the dots and at the eye of the observer merges to form additive mixtures.

COLOR APPEARANCE

For the normal observer, as the wavelength of light is increased from 400 to 700 nm, hues change from violet, to blue, to green, to yellow, to orange, to red. Purples (as opposed to spectral violet) cannot be produced by the presentation of a single wavelength. Purple is obtained by adding together light from the long- and short-wave portions of the spectrum (red and blue). Of the myriad of color sensations, those perceived as homogeneous are blue, green, yellow, and red. These perceptually unique colors are the four so-called primal (or primary) hues.[4]

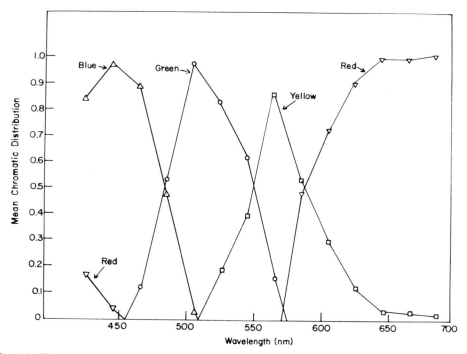

Fig. 5-6. Hue-wavelength correlation obtained with a continuous hue estimation technique. (Data of Smith, V. C., Pokorny, J., and Swartley, R.: Amer. J. Psychol. In press.)

Color naming

Under conditions called neutral adaptation,[5] a hue-wavelength correlation may be obtained. Wavelengths sampled at 10-nm intervals throughout the visible spectrum are presented as brief flashes in random order. The observer is asked to estimate the relative amounts of each of the primal colors for each flash. By averaging a number of presentations at each wavelength a representative hue-wavelength correlation may be obtained (Fig. 5-6). Observers with normal color vision show general agreement in assigning such color names. From the short wavelength end of the spectrum to about 440 nm both the red and blue hues are seen. From about 440 to 530 nm, blue and green hues are present. Between 530 and 570 nm, green and yellow are reported, and beyond 570 nm yellow and red are seen. The regions of overlap occasionally seen between red and green (at 440 and 570 nm) and yellow and blue (at 530 nm) result from the observer on different trials identifying the predominant color as having different secondary components (for example, on different trials 440 nm might be identified as a slightly reddish blue or as a slightly greenish blue).

The spectral locus of a primary hue may be obtained by noting the wavelength at which the two neighboring hues are minimal. By this criterion, blue is associated with wavelengths in the region of 460 nm; green, 505 nm; and yellow, 570 nm. Red does not have a unique spectrum locus; in fact, for most observers primal red results from the mixture of a small amount of blue with long wavelength light.[6]

It is worth noting that each of the primary hues will blend with only two of the other three. For example, red and blue mixtures appear purple and red and yellow mixtures appear orange; but the hue sensations red and green never appear simultaneously in a single percept. There is no such hue as a reddish-green or a greenish-red. Similarly, blue and yellow are never simultaneously perceived. Such pairs of colors (known as complementary colors), when added together, produce the sensation of white.

Color contrast

Color appearances of chromatic stimuli are very sensitive to the conditions of presentation.[7] For example, suppose a circle of 575-nm light is presented both within a white surround area and a red surround area. The 575 nm will appear greenish when it occurs within the red surround and yellow when it occurs within the white surround. A white area presented within a yellow surround will appear tinged with blue. These are examples of simultaneous color contrast. Simultaneous color contrast refers to a change in the appearance of a field as a result of the introduction of a second chromatic stimulus. Change in color appearance of a field produced by preadapting with a chromatic stimulus is called "successive contrast."

Bezold-Brücke and Abney phenomena

Color appearance is affected by interactions of saturation and brightness with hue. Two important phenomena, named after the scientists who first described them, are the Bezold-Brücke and Abney effects, which result from interactions of hue with luminance and saturation respectively.

The Bezold-Brücke phenomenon refers to the fact that only three hues associated with spectral wavelengths appear the same when luminance is changed. For example, a hue associated with 600 nm (orange) appears reddish orange at low luminances and yellowish orange at high luminances. The three hues that do not change are called the invariant hues. They are a blue of about 478 nm, a green of about 503 nm, and a yellow of about 578 nm.[8] These spectral invariants are close to the psychological primary colors (unique hues). A general description of the Bezold-Brücke phenomenon is: at low luminances hues correlated with wavelengths 470 to 578 nm (blue-greens, greens, and yellow-greens) tend to appear greener, while hues correlated with wavelengths above 578 nm (oranges and reds) tend to appear redder than at an intermediate luminance. At a higher luminance, hues correlated with wavelengths below 500 nm (blues and blue-greens) appear bluer and hues correlated with wavelengths above 500 nm (yellow-greens, yellows, and reds) appear yellower than at an intermediate luminance.

The Abney effect refers to the fact that when a hue associated with a spectral wavelength is desaturated by adding a small amount of white, the apparent hue will change.[1] Thus a green associated with 530 nm will appear yellower when white is added to the 530-nm stimulus. There is one exception in the spectral region: a yellow of 570 nm appears invariant with change in saturation. A general description of the Abney effect is: hues correlated with spectral wavelengths between 400 and 570 nm appear like hues associated with longer wavelengths (blue-greens appear greener, yellow-greens appear yellower), while hues associated with wavelengths above 570 nm appear like hues associated with shorter wavelengths (oranges and reds appear yellower). The size of the Abney effect (that is, the apparent hue shift) is variable from wavelength to wavelength.

SPECTRAL SENSITIVITY

The human eye is not equally sensitive to all wavelengths of light. For example, 0.001 watt of radiation at 550 nm (green) appears as a bright light, whereas 0.001 watt of radiation at 450 nm (blue) appears dim.

Threshold measurements

It is important to know the relative energies at which the various wavelengths of light have an equal effect upon the eye. One method is to obtain the absolute threshold response, or least energy at which the presence of a monochromatic test light is detectable on a criterion percentage of trials.[9] The following presents a prototypical experiment to indicate the relevant parameters and how they are controlled. A test light of specified size and duration is used; for example, a circle subtending 40 minutes visual angle is flashed for 20 msec. The subject stays in the dark for 10 to 15 minutes before the experiment begins. The subject is asked to report when he sees the flash, as the energy in the test light is varied. The light is flashed centered entirely within the rod-free fovea where cone density is greatest. The energy required to elicit a response at the visual threshold is greatest in the short- and long-wave ends of the spectrum and is at a minimum at about 550 nm.

At or just above the visual threshold the hue will be identified.[10] A further increase in energy leads to an increase in both apparent brightness and saturation of the hue.[11] The saturation reaches a maximum (at a different energy for each wavelength) and finally at very high (glare) light levels the saturation appears decreased.

Photochromatic interval

For retinal areas outside the fovea, a cone response is obtained at higher energies than for the absolute threshold for the rods whose spectral minimum is at 507 nm (see Chapter 3). For such an extrafoveal test light, as the energy is raised from a minimum value a dim gray is seen first (rods). With a further increase in energy the gray increases in brightness until the cone threshold is reached, at which point a hue may be identified. The interval between the appearance of the achromatic rod response and the chromatic cone response is known as the "photochromatic interval." The transition from rod to cone vision is not abrupt and depends on many factors. The fact that the rod and cone systems have different spectral minima means that a change in illumination near the rod-cone transition level results in a shift in the relative brightness of different portions of the spectrum. This shift is called the Purkinje shift, since it was Purkinje who first noted that as dawn approached, red and yellow flowers (whose dominant reflectance was at wavelengths of 530 nm or longer) would suddenly become brighter than blue flowers and green leaves (whose dominant reflectance was at wavelengths below or close to 507 nm).[12] Further information on the interplay of the responses of rods and cones can be found in Chapter 3.

A problem with using the absolute threshold technique for photopic functions is that since the rod system is more sensitive, an observer can often see a test light merely by shifting his gaze so that the stimulus is no longer on the fovea. Thus, careful fixation is required or the obtained values will be contaminated by rod responses, especially in the short wavelength end of the spectrum.

Spectral sensitivity function

Frequently, data are expressed in terms of sensitivity rather than energy: the greater the sensitivity to a given wavelength, the less energy is required to see at that wavelength. The function obtained by plotting the reciprocal of energy at the threshold against wavelength is called a "spectral sensitivity function."

Spectral sensitivity functions may also be obtained by determining the just-perceptible increment radiance of a monochromatic stimulus flashed on a white

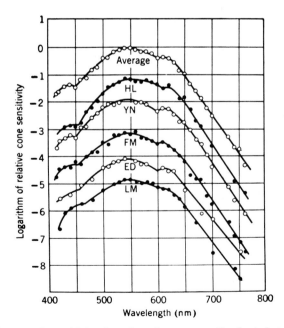

Fig. 5-7. Threshold spectral sensitivity functions for a centrally fixated target. The stimulus was a 42-minute circular target exposed for 4 msec. The upper curve shows the averaged data for the five subjects. For clarity, each successive individual curve has been lowered one logarithmic unit. (After Hsia, Y., and Graham, C. H.: Proc. Nat. Acad. Sci. **38**:83, 1952.)

background field. This technique avoids problems of rod contamination and gives a function generally similar in shape to that obtained at absolute threshold.[13] The major differences are a tendency for depression in long-wave sensitivity and accentuation of irregularities in the spectral sensitivity curve. Both these factors depend on the spectral composition and intensity of the white background.

The spectral sensitivity functions obtained from a given individual are repeatable from day to day, with variability of 0.1 to 0.2 log unit. Differences between observers are of the order of 0.1 to 0.3 log unit. The individual function may show irregularities or bumps, many of which are reproducible both within and between observers.[14] These bumps depend somewhat on experimental conditions, being more obvious when functions are obtained in laboratories using small test fields and extremely monochromatic light. Further, the bumps may be accentuated by the use of high-intensity backgrounds. Fig. 5-7 shows some functions obtained with a test light subtending 42 minutes of arc, flashed for 4 msec. The subjects were dark-adapted and the technique was the method of absolute threshold. Shoulders occur in the curves at 460 nm and 610 to 620 nm. It should be noted that the maximum of the average function has been placed at unity and that the individual functions show variability of 0.3 log unit in the height of their maxima.

Suprathreshold measurements

A different type of methodology used to obtain spectral sensitivity functions is that of matching spectral lights to a reference light. Such techniques include heterochromatic side-by-side matching, cascade matching, and heterochromatic flicker photometry. The obtained functions are often called luminosity functions.

In heterochromatic matching, two test lights are presented side by side at an energy well above the absolute threshold. One test light contains a fixed wavelength, or under certain circumstances white light, and the other a variable wavelength. The subject is asked to match the two test lights in luminance (disregarding any difference in hue). If the hue difference is great, this task is virtually impossible for an observer with normal color vision. For example, very few observers can match a green (530 nm) and a yellow (580 nm) for luminance with any accuracy. Observers are confused by saturation differences and tend to overestimate the luminance of the more highly saturated hues, making luminance matching errors as high as 50%. The method of heterochromatic side-by-side matching, however, can be used successfully for wavelengths 500 to 700 nm when testing persons with sex-linked congenital color defect, since both the apparent saturation and apparent hue difference are reduced for these observers.

A variation of heterochromatic side-by-side matching is the cascade technique. The experimenter starts with a standard wavelength (for example, 550 nm) and a variable wavelength 560 nm (a small hue difference). The observer matches the variable wavelength in luminance to the standard wavelength and the value is noted. Then the experimenter sets the standard wavelength equal to the variable wavelength (both are now at 560 nm) and the observer makes an exact brightness match between the two identical wavelengths. The experimenter sets the variable wavelength at 570 nm (further toward the yellow) and the observer is then ready to make a new match. Thus, in this technique the standard wavelength is constantly changed so that the hue difference between standard and variable wavelength is never great. If care is taken, the cascade technique yields a spectral sensitivity function similar in shape to those obtained using the absolute threshold technique, although at a different luminance level. Any small errors in matching, however, are successively compounded.

The third and most common method of obtaining spectral sensitivity functions is the method of heterochromatic flicker photometry. In this method a test wavelength is alternated with a white at a slow rate (10 to 18 cps). The white light is set at a standard brightness above absolute threshold. When the luminance difference between the test and the white is great—that is, the test either brighter or dimmer than the standard white—there is a sensation of flicker, which becomes less apparent as the luminance of the test wavelength approaches that of the white. When the test is equal in luminance to the standard, the sensation

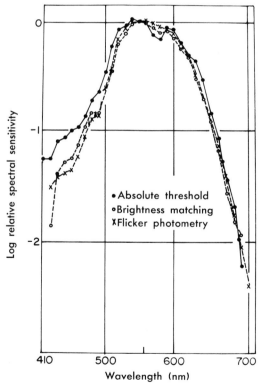

Fig. 5-8. Spectral sensitivity functions using three different methods. The threshold data were obtained with a 45-minute circular target exposed for 4 msec. The brightness matching and flicker photometry data were obtained with a 2-degree field at a retinal illuminance of 500 trolands. Functions plotted represent the average of three observers. (After Sperling, H. G., and Lewis, W. G.: J. Opt. Soc. Amer. **49:**986, 1959.)

of flicker is at a minimum and may be eliminated by an increase in the alternation rate. At slightly higher rates of alternation, the appearance of flicker is eliminated not only at the luminance match but also in a narrow range of luminances close to the match, and the flicker sensation occurs only when a large luminance mismatch exists. Thus, the observer's task consists of adjusting the test wavelength luminance in order to eliminate or minimize the sensation of flicker. By convention, the reciprocal of the relative energy values obtained at a number of wavelengths define the spectral sensitivity function. The heterochromatic flicker technique is the most widely used of the three techniques since it is the fastest and easiest for the subject. Fig. 5-8 shows a comparison of the results of the methods cited.

Of the various methods of measuring spectral sensitivity described, only the absolute threshold method allows for absolute comparisons of sensitivity between individuals. For the other methods, a comparison stimulus is present and the data are expressed in reference to the sensitivity of the observer to this stimulus (for example, a neutral density filter that attenuates the standard and comparison lights 50% would not appreciably alter the sensitivity function obtained using a matching technique; however, such a filter would uniformly displace an absolute threshold function by 0.3 log unit).

Standard Observer

The concept of the Standard Observer was devised by the Committee Intérnationale d'Eclairage (CIE) in order to standardize a photopic sensitivity function for use in photometry and colorimetry. Fig. 5-9 shows the function accepted by the CIE in 1924 and called the CIE relative photopic luminosity function (V_λ). This function represents average data from seven laboratories

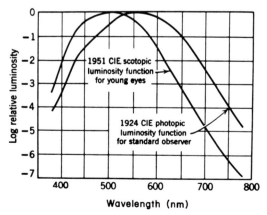

Fig. 5-9. Log relative luminosity for the rods and cones. The curve to the right is the 1924 CIE photopic luminosity V_λ function for the Standard Observer. The curve to the left is the 1951 CIE scotopic luminosity V_λ' function for young eyes. The curves are so adjusted that maximum visibility for each is set at unity. (After Graham, C. H.: Vision and visual perception, New York, 1965, John Wiley & Sons, Inc., p. 353.)

with a total of more than 300 observers. Some of the data are based on the cascade technique and some on the flicker technique of heterochromatic photometry. Recent work suggests that the luminosities in the blue may have been underestimated.[15] Also shown on this figure is the 1951 CIE scotopic luminosity function for young eyes V'_λ. This function is based on absolute threshold data. Both V_λ and V'_λ have been assigned a value of unity at their maximum.

COLORIMETRY

We mentioned earlier that hue is correlated with wavelength, but there are many ways of producing the same hue sensation. For example, a "yellow" can be produced by a monochromatic radiation (590 nm) or by the additive mixture of a green (545 nm) and a red (670 nm). When you look at a yellow object, you have no way of knowing from its appearance the spectral composition of the physical stimulus. The aim of colorimetry is to provide an economical system of color measurement and specification based upon the concept of equivalent-appearing stimuli.

Metamerism

In this section we are going to discuss the results of experiments in which colors are matched by mixing colored lights. Fig. 5-10 shows a typical example

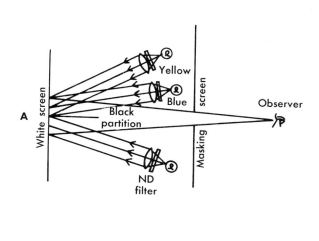

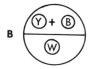

Fig. 5-10. A, Hypothetical representation of a color mixture experiment. The top half of the bipartite field is illuminated by the additive combination of light transmitted by the yellow and blue filters. The bottom half of the field is illuminated by a tungsten filament lamp with a neutral density filter inserted to equate the luminances of the two halves. **B,** View of the field as seen by the observer.

of a color-matching experiment. The two halves of the bipartite field contain dissimilar spectral radiations and yet are seen as the same by the observer. Such pairs of colors are known as metameric pairs or metameric objects. Different observers will use slightly different amounts of the two monochromatic radiations. We can write an equation for this match by taking an average of the matches of many people (Standard Observer). The metameric equation for this match may be represented as:

$$L_B \;(B) + L_Y \;(Y) \equiv L_w \;(W)$$

where the symbol $\equiv$ means "matches," the encircled terms represent the colors, and the terms denoted L represent the quantities of each of the colors used.[3]

A color match is invariant under a variety of experimental conditions that may alter the appearance of the matching fields. If an observer looks at a metameric match to white after preexposure to a moderately bright green field, both halves of the field will appear reddish in hue but will still appear identical. Likewise, if a chromatic surround is placed around the matching fields, simultaneous contrast will change the appearance of the fields but the metamerism still holds. When we speak of specific hues and degrees of saturation with reference to color mixtures, a neutral state of adaptation is assumed.

Complementary colors

There are many pairs of colors that, when added together, match white. Such pairs are known as "complementary colors." Mixtures of yellow and blue, or orange and greenish-blue, or red and blue-green in appropriate proportions all yield equivalent sensations. Table 1 gives a number of experimentally determined pairs of complementary colors and the amounts of each required to match a standard white when each wavelength is set at an equivalent luminance. It should be noted that no complementary colors are specified on the table for

Table 1. Spectral complementaries and proportions to match a unit amount of white in the equation $L_{\lambda 1}(\lambda_1) + L_{\lambda 2}(\lambda_2) \equiv 1.0 \;(W)$ *

$\lambda 1$	$\lambda 2$	$L_{\lambda 2}$	$L_{\lambda 1}$
Extreme red	496.5	42.1	57.9
609	493.5	52.4	47.6
591	490	67.1	32.9
586	487.5	73.9	26.1
580	482.5	82.7	17.3
578.5	480.5	85.6	14.4
576.5	477.5	87.7	12.3
575.5	474.5	90.3	9.7
574	472	92.0	8.0
573	466.5	94.1	5.9
572	459	96.1	3.9
570.5	Extreme violet	97.6	2.4

*Recalculated from data of Sinden, R. H.: J. Opt. Soc. Amer. **7**:1123, 1923. The color temperature of white light is 5,000 K.

the central region of the spectrum from 500 to 560 nm. Green does not have a spectral complement. In order to match a white, some red and some blue must be added together with the green.

$$L_G\widehat{G} + L_R\widehat{R} + L_B\widehat{B} \equiv L_w\widehat{W}$$

Chromaticity diagram

The results of color matching experiments can conveniently be expressed on a color mixture diagram designed so that distances are proportional to the amounts of each color used (Fig. 5-11).

In Fig. 5-11, the hue is represented around the perimeter and the saturation as the distance from the center. Luminance is not represented on the diagram. By drawing a straight line through a spectral color and the point designated as white, the intersection of the line with the other side of the diagram specifies the position of the complementary color. In a similar manner, all color mixtures can be represented by joining the colors being mixed with a straight line on the diagram and specifying the resultant mixture as a point on the line representing the relative amounts of the two colors used.

Algebra of color mixture

The chromaticity diagram shown in Fig. 5-11 was experimentally obtained by determining the amounts of red $\widehat{R}$, green $\widehat{G}$, and blue $\widehat{B}$ primaries required to match spectral stimuli.[16] For example, a blue-green (λ 490) can be matched in hue with an additive mixture of $\widehat{G}$ and $\widehat{B}$, but the spectral blue-green is slightly more saturated than the mixture. The two halves of the matching field can be made to appear identical by adding a small amount of R to the spectral blue-green.

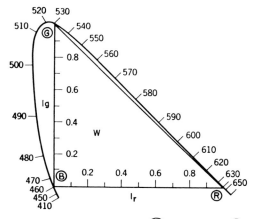

Fig. 5-11. Chromaticity diagram based on primaries $\widehat{B}$ = 460 nm, $\widehat{G}$ = 530 nm, and $\widehat{R}$ = 650 nm. (After Wright, W. D.: Researches on normal and defective colour vision, London, 1946, Henry Kimpton.)

$$L_{490}\,\text{\textcircled{490}} + L_{R}\text{\textcircled{R}} \equiv L_{G}\text{\textcircled{G}} + L_{B}\text{\textcircled{B}}$$

If we wish to express the spectral blue-green in terms of the three primaries, we can treat this as an equation and say:

$$L_{490}\,\text{\textcircled{490}} \equiv L_{G}\text{\textcircled{G}} + L_{B}\text{\textcircled{B}} - L_{R}\text{\textcircled{R}}$$

L_R, L_G, and L_B are called the tristimulus values and they represent the amounts of the primaries $\text{\textcircled{R}}$, $\text{\textcircled{G}}$, and $\text{\textcircled{B}}$.

In a similar manner, every point on the chromaticity diagrams (that is, every seen color) can be specified in terms of three primaries, with one of the three sometimes being negative. What does a negative amount mean? It means only that the mixture of the two positive primaries is not as saturated as the color to be matched.

Let's look a little more closely at the manner in which the diagram is set up. The distance along the abscissa represents the proportion of the red primary. The distance along the ordinate represents the proportion of the green primary. The amount of the blue primary is determined by noting the difference between the sum of the red and green and the total. To do this conveniently, the tristimulus values are converted into a form where the sum of the three always equals unity.

$$l_r = \frac{L_R}{L_R + L_G + L_B} \qquad l_g = \frac{L_G}{L_R + L_G + L_B} \qquad l_b = \frac{L_B}{L_R + L_G + L_B}$$

The coefficients l_r, l_g, and l_b sum to unity and are called the chromaticity coordinates or trichromatic coefficients. If l_r is plotted against l_g, an isosceles right-angle triangle results within which all points can be specified in terms of the three chromaticity coordinates. The bowing in Fig. 5-11 represents the negative values that the primaries take on in the specification of the spectral colors. l_r is slightly negative for the spectral region ranging from blue to green, and l_b is slightly negative for the spectral region including green, yellow, and red. The values of $\text{\textcircled{B}}$, $\text{\textcircled{G}}$, and $\text{\textcircled{R}}$ are determined by a logic and design of a given experiment. In Table 1 they are given by the luminance of each wavelength. In Fig. 5-11 they represent the setting of L_G and L_R equal at 582.5 nm and L_B and L_G equal at 494 nm, a procedure that eliminates intrasubject variability for spectral colors caused by nonreceptoral absorption characteristics.[16]

This discussion is based on three arbitrarily chosen primaries. In fact, there are many sets of primaries that can be used. The only restriction is that no primary may be matched in hue by a combination of the other two primaries.[15] Likewise, other chromaticity systems and diagrams can be algebraically derived from the original set of primaries.[17,18]

XYZ system

Although in actual practice one of the three primaries is usually negative (presumably because all spectral lights stimulate to some degree more than one photopigment), it is possible by algebraic manipulation to devise a system in which all values of the three primaries for all mixtures are positive. Fig. 5-12 shows the chromaticity diagram derived for the XYZ system.[15] It was set up

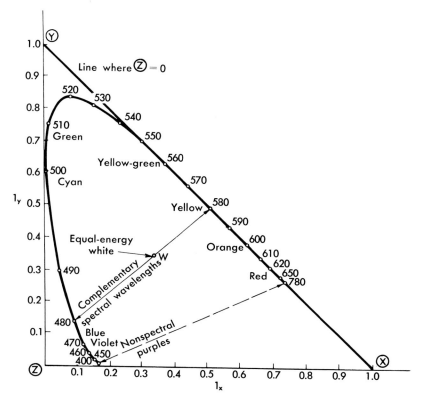

Fig. 5-12. XYZ chromaticity diagram. The three primaries, *X, Y,* and *Z* are imaginary (that is, not experimentally realizable). All computations utilizing this diagram involve positive numbers (the spectrum locus is entirely contained within the triangle *XYZ*). (After Boynton, R. M. In Sidowski, J. B., editor: Experimental methods and instrumentation in psychology, New York, 1966, McGraw-Hill Book Co., p. 296.)

to satisfy the criteria that there be no negative numbers and that the tristimulus values of Y for the spectrum be those of V_λ (CIE photopic luminosity function for the Standard Observer). The primaries X, Y, and Z are called "imaginary primaries." They lie outside the experimentally determined chromaticity diagram and can be thought of as being more saturated than spectral colors.

COLOR DISCRIMINATIONS
Wavelength discrimination

Wavelength discrimination refers to the ability of an observer to detect differences in wavelength. In a representative wavelength discrimination experiment, the observer views two fields, one filled with light of a standard wavelength (that is, a narrow spectral band of light) and the other with light of a comparison wavelength. Initially, both fields contain the same wavelength. The wavelength of the comparison field is changed in small steps (1 nm or less) until the observer reports that the fields do not appear the same hue. It is important

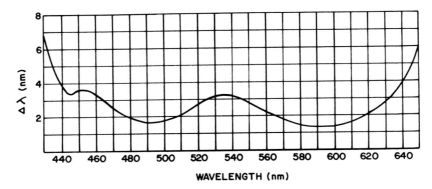

Fig. 5-13. Wavelength discrimination function obtained by Wright and Pitt (Proc. Phys. Soc. [London] **46**:463, 1934). The just-discriminable wavelength step (△λ) is plotted against wavelength. The function represents the average data from five observers.

to adjust the luminance of the comparison field to maintain both fields of equal luminance so that the discrimination is not made on the basis of a brightness difference.[16] The size of the wavelength difference at which the observer reports a hue difference is called the "wavelength discrimination step" (delta lambda) and the procedure is repeated for many standard wavelengths in the visible spectrum. Fig. 5-13 presents a wavelength discrimination function showing the value of delta lambda as a function of the standard wavelength. The function shows a number of peaks and valleys and the scale is of the order of 1 to 6 nm. Relative minima occur in the yellow (590 nm), blue-green (490 nm), and blue (440 nm); relative maxima occur in the blue (450 nm) and green (530 nm). At the ends of the spectrum in the deep blue (below 430 nm) and far red (above 650 nm) wavelength discrimination deteriorates rapidly.

In an alternative procedure the experimenter initially sets the two fields to be different in wavelength. The observer is asked to adjust the variable wavelength until the fields appear the same. The measure of discrimination is taken as the standard deviation of the matching wavelengths.[19]

Saturation and colorimetric purity

Saturation refers to the "paleness" or "whiteness" of a color. A non-spectral color such as pink may be specified as a mixture of red and white. We may think of a series of such mixtures ranging from white through pink to red, each of which has the same dominant wavelength and is of the same brightness, differing only in the ratio of monochromatic spectral red to white. An observer can arrange such color mixtures in an orderly sequence from white to red, and we would say that the colors vary in their saturation. Adding white to a color desaturates that color. The term "colorimetric purity," p, has been defined for such mixtures as the ratio $p = L_\lambda / L_w + L_\lambda$ where L_λ is the luminance of the spectral color and L_w is the luminance of white. The value of p varies between 0 for a white and 1.0 for a spectral radiation.

Although this definition of colorimetric purity assigns a value of unity to all

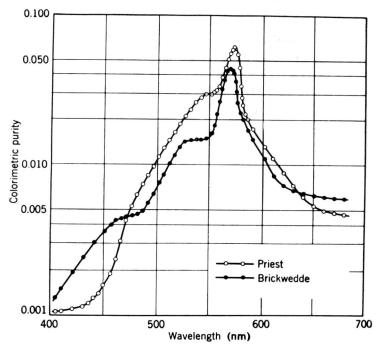

Fig. 5-14. Least colorimetric purity as a function of wavelength. (Data of Priest, I. G., and Brick-wedde, F. G.: J. Opt. Soc. Amer. **28:**133-139, 1938, as shown by Hecht, S. In Merchison, C., editor: A handbook of general experimental psychology, Worcester, 1934, Clark University Press, p. 801.)

spectral radiations, the spectral colors do not appear equally saturated. A spectral blue (450 nm) appears more saturated than a spectral yellow (580 nm) of equal brightness. An index of saturation for different wavelengths is obtained from the data of an experiment that determines least colorimetric purity for successive wavelengths, that is, the just-discriminable difference between two fields differing only in saturation. For such determinations, the standard field is white and the variable field contains a mixture of white plus a spectral wavelength. The experimenter increases the proportion of L_λ to L_W in the variable field, maintaining the luminance ($L_\lambda + L_W$) constant and equal to the standard field. The observer reports when the fields first appear different, that is, when the variable field is perceptibly tinged with color.

Fig. 5-14 shows the results of such an experiment. The lowest value of least colorimetric purity occurs in the blue, increasing steadily to a maximum value in the yellow and then decreasing again in the red. The index of saturation is the reciprocal of the least colorimetric purity. The colors with the greatest saturation—blues and reds—are those for which only a small amount of L_λ is necessary to make a white appear tinged with color. Similarly, successive purity discriminations can be obtained, for example, a pink from a reddish-pink. Such experiments indicate that there are more discriminable steps between white and the spectral radiation for the highly saturated hues (blues and reds) than there are for the less saturated hues (yellows).[20]

A color may also be desaturated by increasing its spectral half width or by adding a small amount of the complementary wavelength while maintaining the same dominant wavelength and total luminance. Similarly, hues obtained by the mixing of two spectral wavelengths are desaturated with respect to the matching dominant wavelength.

MECHANISM OF COLOR VISION
Trichromatic and opponent-process theories

Historically, two pretheoretical ideas have dominated color theory. First, the trivariance of vision, as exemplified by the data of color mixture, suggested that there might be three fundamental sensation curves. A theory based on this hypothesis is called a trichromatic theory. Many theorists have thought that the spectral sensitivity of the fundamental sensation curves are determined by cone receptor photopigments. Second, certain perceptual phenomena, such as contrast, and the observation that when complementary colors are added together the chromatic qualities cancel each other suggested the hypothesis that nervous elements may respond in a bivariant manner, giving one sort of response in a given spectral region and an opposite response in another spectral region. This is the basis of the opponent-process theory. A zone or stage theory combines aspects of both the trichromatic and opponent-process theories.

Current evidence indicates that the trichromatic approach seems valid in terms of the photopigments that absorb light. Electrophysiological experiments indicate that this trivariant information is transformed and transmitted in an opponent process manner in the nervous system.

Spectral response of the three pigments: psychophysical approaches

Thomas Young in 1802[21] suggested that the eye need only have three independent modes of excitation with each of these being differentially sensitive in the visible spectrum and having peak sensitivities in different regions of the spectrum.

Early attempts to discover the spectral response of cone pigments involved psychophysical studies designed to isolate one of the receptor mechanisms. One class of experiment is the bleaching experiment, in which the observer is adapted to an intense spectral light, following which matching equations or relative spectral sensitivity thresholds are obtained. If, for example, a 650-nm light is used for the bleach, it is hypothesized that the long wavelength receptor mechanism is bleached more than the middle or short wavelength receptor mechanisms. Thus, the observer's matches or thresholds after a red bleach should reflect primarily the activities of the middle or short wavelength receptors. This technique has limitations, since the receptor sensitivities are very close and any bleaching light tends to adapt all the mechanisms. The technique is most successful when long wavelength bleaching lights are used to isolate the short and middle wavelength receptor mechanisms.

A second class of experiment is the two-color threshold. In 1939 Stiles[22] reported a series of experiments from which he was able to deduce five independent chromatic mechanisms, which he labeled $\pi_1 - \pi_5$. Stiles' technique was to measure increment thresholds (that is, the least perceptible radiance increment of a flash presented on a background field) using different wavelengths for test and background. The rationale for the technique such as in the bleaching experiments is that by suitable choice of the background wavelength it is possible to adapt differentially the different receptor mechanisms. The technique has the advantage that even when there are only small differences in sensitivity between two or three mechanisms, their increment threshold responses may still be independently recognized as the background radiance is changed. For example, with a 540-nm background and a 480-nm test flash, the increment thresholds are determined by the Stiles π_4 (middle wavelength) mechanism at threshold and low radiances of background and by the Stiles π_1 (short wavelength) mechanism at higher radiances of background. It is now recognized that the π mechanisms do not represent the responses of isolated pigments.

A third class of experiment is that in which observers with reduced color vision systems are used as observers. For example, the protanope is an observer who is presumed to be missing the long wavelength receptor mechanism. Absolute threshold spectral sensitivity obtained on a protanope thus reflects activity only of the short and middle wavelength mechanisms. Since there is evidence that the short wavelength receptors contribute only in a minor way to luminosity, the protanope's spectral sensitivity reflects mainly activity of the middle wavelength receptor. Similarly, the spectral sensitivity of a deuteranopic observer should reflect primarily the activity of the long wavelength receptor. A very rare type of observer, the blue monocone monochromat, allows direct measurement of the spectral response of the short wavelength receptor mechanism. This observer appears in many respects like a rod monochromat, but he does have normal short wavelength–sensitive cones. At high photopic levels of illumination, only these blue cones are active and the observer's spectral sensitivity function is that of the short wavelength mechanism.

Direct measurement of cone pigments

In recent years there have been attempts to measure the cone pigments directly. Rushton[23] applied the technique of retinal densitometry to measuring the foveal response of normal observers, protanopes, and deuteranopes. In retinal densitometry a bright light is shone into the eye and measurements are made of that portion of the light reflected back out of the eye. The reflected light has suffered attenuation by absorbance in the ocular media, neural structures, and pigments themselves. When a bleaching light is used, measurements may be made of the change in reflectance (pre- and postbleaching) of various wavelengths. The resulting function is called a difference spectrum. Rushton discovered two pigments, a long wavelength–absorbing pigment, which he called erytholabe, and a middle wavelength–absorbing pigment, which he called chlorolabe. He did not detect a short wavelength–sensitive pigment. Chlorolabe was the sole pigment found in the protanope. This pigment could be demonstrated in the normal observer by the method of partial bleaching, in which a long-wave light is used for bleaching. Erytholabe, also found in the normal by partial bleaching, could be demonstrated as the sole pigment of the deuteranopic subject. Rushton's data show considerable variability but have the same shape as the psychophysical data. Their importance lies in the fact that Rushton's data are the first to demonstrate objectively that protanopes and deuteranopes are each missing one of the normal cone photopigments.

There are reports from two laboratories that have succeeded in making spectrophotometric measurements on isolated cones from monkey and human retinas. In this technique, light is transmitted through single cones or sections of retina containing cones. A light-sensitive photocell placed behind the cone compares transmission for each wavelength for the beam passing through the cone and a reference beam. A white light bleach may be used in order to obtain difference spectra. This is an extremely difficult undertaking, since the cone outer segments are small and the pigments absorb only a small percentage of the incident light. In addition, the measuring light itself bleaches the pigment during the course of the experiment.

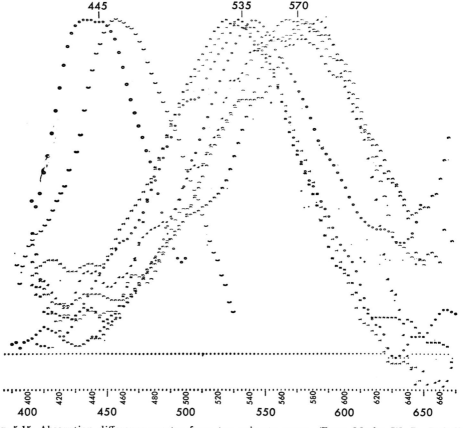

Fig. 5-15. Absorption difference spectra from ten primate cones. (From Marks, W. B., Dobelle, W. H., and MacNichol, E. F.: Science **143**:1182, 1964.)

Marks, Dobelle, and MacNichol[24] were able to obtain recordings from ten primate cones, Brown and Wald[25] from four human cones. The difference spectra of these individual cones show a maximum change of absorbance of .02. Their wavelengths of peak sensitivity are quite variable. Fig. 5-15 shows some results from MacNichol's laboratory. The cones appear to group in three classes with peak sensitivity at 565, 535, and 445 nm. Both laboratories have reported extreme difficulty in locating and measuring the short wavelength–sensitive cones.

Comparison of results

Fig. 5-16 shows a comparison of the hypothesized spectral response of the three classes of cones as obtained by psychophysical techniques and by direct measurements of bleaching. The solid lines fitted to the various sets of data represent a transformation of the CIE color matching data.

There is good general agreement between data collected with a variety of techniques. These data thus provide a solid foundation for the hypothesis that human color vision is mediated by three classes of cone pigment, whose maximal sensitivities occur at about 435, 535, and 560 nm, respectively.

Psychophysical evidence for opponent-process mode of neural processing

Although many of the phenomena of color vision can be explained within the trichromatic framework, certain perceptions are more economically and intuitively explained with reference to an opponent-process schema. For example, there are four perceptually unique colors: red, yellow, green, and blue. Why should a system based upon three types of receptors produce four unique types of sensations? The other general class of data that seems difficult to place intuitively within the trichromatic framework involves a variety of conditions under which the visual system seems to function in terms of pairs of colors. Complementary colors, when added together, produce an achromatic sensation, white. The negative after-image is complementary to the physical stimulus. If an observer stares at a chromatic stimulus for an extended period of time and then shifts gaze to a white surface, the color sensation of the after-image projected on the white surface is that of the complement of the inducing chromatic stimulus.

Phenomena such as these led Hering in the late 1800's to propose an opponent-process theory. He considered yellow as a primary color along with red, green, and blue. Based upon the complementary nature of blue and yellow and red and green, Hering suggested that these four colors, together with black and white, form three pairs of unique sensory qualities. Further, since the members of each pair are never simultaneously perceived in a single hue percept, the two are considered as mutually exclusive or opponent sensory qualities.

These ideas were disregarded by many scientists because they did not conform to their current knowledge of visual physiology. Hurvich and Jameson in the mid-1950's revised Hering's notions with the publication of a modern opponent-process theory.[26] Using a psychophysical technique, they obtained responses purported to represent the activity of an opponent-process mechanism. Their basic technique involved the presentation of a spectral wavelength mixed with one of the four primal hues, red, green, yellow, and blue. The subject's task was to increase the energy of the primal stimulus until no trace of its complement occurred in the mixture. For example, suppose a blue-green is mixed with primal yellow; as the ratio of yellow to blue-green increases, the appearance of the mixture varies from blue-green, to desaturated green, to yellow. The experimenter is interested in knowing the minimum amount of yellow necessary to

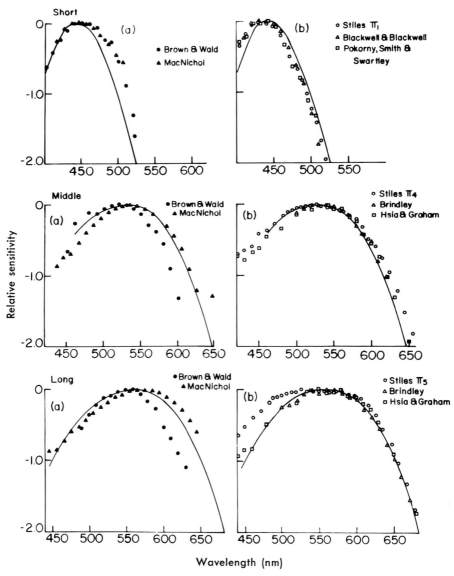

Fig. 5-16. For legend see opposite page.

cancel the blue and give a green-appearing mixture. At the same blue-green wavelength, red can be added and the amount of red necessary to cancel the green may be obtained. The procedure is repeated for all spectral wavelengths and chromatic valence curves of the type shown in Fig. 5-17 are obtained.

Physiological evidence of opponent-process responses

Physiological confirmation of these types of response patterns were first observed for freshwater fish by Svaetichin and his associates[27] and later in primates by DeValois and his colleagues.[28] DeValois recorded from single units in the lateral geniculate nucleus of the macaque monkey. In the absence of a visual stimulus, cells are spontaneously active, that is, they exhibit a random pattern of spike firing. When a spectral stimulus is flashed, there are three possible response patterns: the cell may respond with an increased firing rate to all wavelengths (excitators), with decreased firing rate to all wavelengths (inhibitors), or with increased firing rate to some wavelengths and a decreased firing rate to others (spectrally opponent). Of the cells sampled, about one-third were either excitators or inhibitors and the remaining two-thirds were spectrally opponent. Fig. 5-18 shows a comparison between the excitators and the normal human spectral sensitivity function, and Fig. 5-19 shows the spectrally opponent cells, which fall into four categories: The +B−Y cells increase in firing rate when short-wave light is flashed and decrease in rate when long-wave light is flashed. +Y−B cells (not shown on graph) are observed with about equal frequency. These cells are essentially a mirror image of the +B−Y cells, showing increased firing for yellow and decreased firing for blue. The two other types of cells, +R−G and +G−R, show spectrally opponent behavior over a different portion of the spectrum. Again there is good general agreement between the psychophysical data of man and electrophysiological data of monkeys. Data of this sort have placed the opponent-process theory on a sound physiological basis.

Fig. 5-16. Comparison of a number of attempts to specify the human cone receptor mechanisms. (a), Microspectrophotometric difference spectra from individual cones. The solid curves are explained in the text. (Data of Brown, P. K., and Wald, G.: Science **144**:145-151, 1964, and Marks, W. B., Dobelle, W. H., and MacNichol, E. F.: Science **143**:1181-1183, 1964; average of their best records from MacNichol, E. F.: Proc. Nat. Acad. Sci. **55**:1336, 1966.) (b), Psychophysical determinations of special sensitivities of the color mechanisms. For the short wavelength pigment, Stiles π_1 function is a theoretical function derived from increment threshold studies using color normal observers. (Data tabulated in Wyszecki, G., and Stiles, W. S.: Color science, New York, 1967, John Wiley & Sons, Inc., p. 579.) The other two functions are direct measurements of the sensitivity of persons deficient in both long and middle wavelength sensitive cones (blue monocone monochromat, extremely rare). (Data of Blackwell, R., and Blackwell, O.: Vis. Res. **1**:77, 1961, and Pokorny, J., Smith, V. C., and Swartley, R.: Invest. Ophthal. **9**:809, 1970.) For the middle and long wavelength receptor spectral sensitivity functions, Stiles π functions are derived from increment threshold data using color normal observers. Neither are now believed to represent an isolated cone pigment. Brindley's data (J. Physiol. **122**:338, 1953) are from measurements of spectral sensitivity after intense spectral bleaches using color normals. Hsia and Graham's determinations (Proc. Nat. Acad. Sci. **43**:1017, 1957) are of the spectral sensitivities of protanopes and deuteranopes. Data have been corrected for the absorption characteristics of the lens and macular pigment. Solid curves are described in the text.

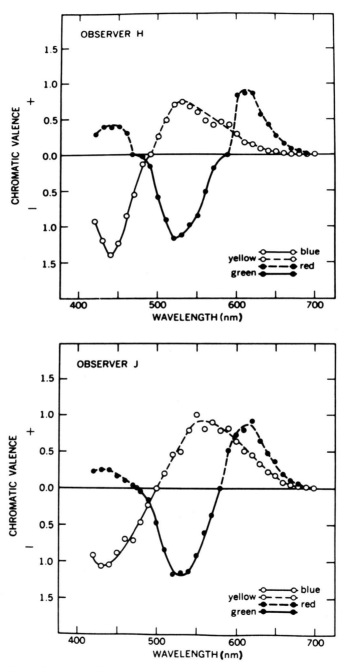

Fig. 5-17. Experimentally determined chromatic valence functions for two observers. (After Jameson, D., and Hurvich, L. M.: J. Opt. Soc. Amer. **45**:550-551, 1955.)

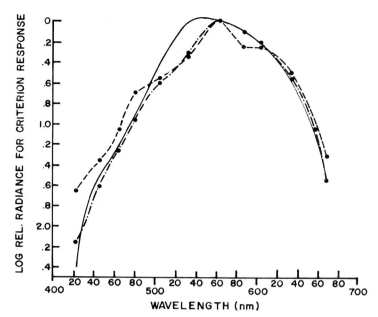

Fig. 5-18. Equal-response spectral sensitivity functions (response criteria): ●— —●, fourteen spikes per second; ●—•—●, eighteen spikes per second for nonopponent excitatory cells compared with the CIE photopic luminosity function (—). (From DeValois, R., Abramov, I., and Jacobs, G. H.: J. Opt. Soc. Amer. **56**:974, 1966.)

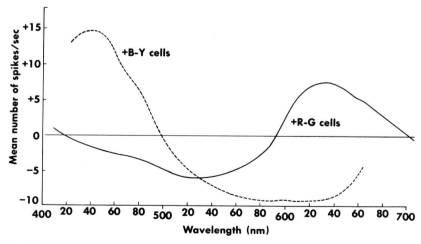

Fig. 5-19. Mean spectral response curves for an equal energy spectrum for +B—Y and +R—G cells. In addition, there are +Y—B and +G—R cells. The curves have been corrected for a spontaneous rate. (From Newell, F. W.: Ophthalmology, principles and concepts, St. Louis, 1969, The C. V. Mosby Co.; after DeValois, R., Abramov, I., and Jacobs, G. H.: J. Opt. Soc. Amer. **56**: 972, 1966.)

Conclusions

Current theories of the color mechanism hypothesize three classes of receptors with three photopigments exhibiting maxima near 435, 535, and 560 nm. The outputs of these receptors (directly or indirectly) may be either excitatory or inhibitory in their effect on higher order neurons, thus allowing for mutually antagonistic responses.

In conclusion, it may be noted that the essentials of our present notions of color mechanism were well understood by Young, Helmholtz, Maxwell, and Hering. Current research in color vision emphasizes the continuing attempt to specify the exact nature of the visual pigments and of the interactions among the chromatic mechanisms.

REFERENCES

1. Wyszecki, G., and Stiles, W. S.: Color science: concepts and methods, quantitative data and formulas, New York, 1967, John Wiley & Sons, Inc.
2. Boynton, R. M.: Vision. In Sidowski, J. B., editor: Experimental methods and instrumentation in psychology, New York, 1966, McGraw-Hill Book Co.
3. Billmeyer, F. W., and Saltzman, M.: Principles of color technology, New York, 1966, John Wiley & Sons, Inc.
4. Linksz, A.: An essay on color vision, New York, 1964, Grune and Stratton, Inc.
5. Hurvich, L. M., and Jameson, D.: A psychophysical study of white, I, III, J. Opt. Soc. Amer. 41:521, 787, 1951; Jameson, D., and Hurvich, L. M.: A psychophysical study of white, II, J. Opt. Soc. Amer. 41:528, 1951.
6. Southall, J. P. C.: Introduction to physiological optics, Oxford, 1937, Oxford University Press.
7. Jameson, D., and Hurvich, L. M.: Perceived color and its dependence on local, surrounding, and preceding stimulus variables, J. Opt. Soc. Amer. 49:890, 1959.
8. Purdy, D. M.: The Bezold-Brücke phenomenon and contours for constant hue, Amer. J. Psychol. 49:313, 1937.
9. Hsia, Y., and Graham, C. H.: Spectral sensitivity of the cones in the dark adapted human eye, Proc. Nat. Acad. Sci. 38:80, 1952.
10. Graham, C. H., and Hsia, Y.: Saturation and the foveal achromatic interval, J. Opt. Soc. Amer. 59:993, 1969.
11. Dagher, M., Cruz, A., and LaPlaza, L.: Colour thresholds with monochromatic stimuli in spectral region 530-630 mμ. In Visual problems of colour, New York, 1961, Chemical Publishing Co.
12. von Helmholtz, H.: Treatise on physiological optics, vol. II (translated by J. P. C. Southall), Rochester, N. Y., 1924, Optical Society of America.
13. Sperling, G., and Lewis, W. G.: Some comparisons between foveal spectral sensitivity data obtained at high brightness and absolute threshold, J. Opt. Soc. Amer. 49:983, 1959.
14. Sheppard, J. J.: Human color perception, New York, 1968, American Elsevier Co.
15. Graham, C. H., editor: Vision and visual perception, New York, 1965, John Wiley & Sons, Inc.
16. Wright, W. D.: Researches on normal and defective colour vision, London, 1946, Henry Kimpton.
17. Le Grand, Y.: Light, colour, and vision, ed. 2 (translated by R. W. G. Hunt, J. W. T. Walsh, and F. R. W. Hunt), London, 1968, Chapman and Hall Ltd.
18. Wright, W. D.: The measurement of colour, ed. 3, London, 1964, Hilger and Watts.
19. MacAdam, D. L.: Visual sensitivities to color differences in daylight, J. Opt. Soc. Amer. 32:247, 1942.
20. Martin, L. C., Warburton, F. L., and Morgan, W. J.: The determination of the sensitiveness of the eye to differences in the saturation of colours, Med. Res. Council Rep. (London) 188:1, 1933.

21. Young, T.: On the theory of light and colors. In MacAdam, D. L., editor: Sources of color science, Cambridge, Mass., 1970, MIT Press.
22. Stiles, W. S.: The directional sensitivity of the retina and the spectral sensitivities of the rods and cones, Proc. Roy. Soc. (London) **127B:**64, 1939.
23. Rushton, W. A. H.: Color vision: an approach through the cones, Invest. Ophthal. **10:**311, 1971.
24. Marks, W. B., Dobelle, W. H., and MacNichol, E. F.: Visual pigments of single primate cones, Science **143:**1181, 1964.
25. Brown, P. K., and Wald, G.: Visual pigments in single rods and cones of the human retina, Science **144:**45, 1964.
26. Hurvich, L. M., and Jameson, D.: An opponent-process theory of color vision, Psychol. Rev. **64:**384, 1957.
27. Svaetichin, G., Negichi, K., and Fatehchand, R.: Cellular mechanisms of Young-Hering visual system. In de Reuck, A. V. S., and Knight, J., editors: CIBA Foundation Symposium: Colour vision, Boston, 1965, Little, Brown and Co.
28. De Valois, R. L., Abramov, I., and Jacobs, G. H.: Analysis of response patterns of LGN cells, J. Opt. Soc. Amer. **56:**966, 1966.

CHAPTER *6* *Abnormal color vision*

ALEX E. KRILL

TYPES OF COLOR BLINDNESS

The nomenclature of congenital color vision defects is derived from the classical concept that there are three fundamental colors, red, green, and blue, called respectively the first, second, and third primaries. By convention, the Greek words for first, second, and third (*protos, deuteros,* and *tritos*) are substituted for red, green, and blue in naming partial color defects. (See outline below.) For example, any word for a red defect has the prefix "proto-."

  I. Trichromat
    A. Normal
    B. Protanomaly
    C. Deuteranomaly
    D. Tritanomaly

 II. Dichromat
    A. Protanopia
    B. Deuteranopia
    C. Tritanopia

III. Monochromat
    A. Rod monochromat
    B. Cone monochromat

The suffix indicates whether there is thought to be a complete absence of the pigment (-anopia), whether the pigment is present but abnormal in some way (-anomaly), or whether the pigment is abnormal in some unspecified way (-an). This last category lumps anomals and anopes together.

A normal subject matches all spectral colors with mixtures of three properly chosen colors and is said to have trichromatic color vision. (See outline above.) Subjects performing as if they had a deficiency of one cone pigment are called anomalous trichromats and require more than normal amount of one color in a mixture.* A dichromat performs as if he had an absence of one cone pigment and can match all spectral colors with two properly chosen colors. A monochromat, on the other hand, can match all spectral colors with different bright-

---

*The actual defect may not be a deficiency of the pigment but rather something else, such as an abnormal type of pigment.

Table 2. Incidence and inheritance of color vision defects

Type	Incidence*	Inheritance†
Deuteranomaly	0.05	X-R
Deuteranopia	0.01	X-R
Protanomaly	0.01	X-R
Protanopia	0.01	X-R
Tritanomaly and tritanopia	0.0001-0.0005‡	A-D
Rod monochromatism	0.0003	
Complete		A-R
Incomplete		A-R or X-R
Cone monochromatism	0.00000001	?

*Based on data from Europe and the United States.
†X-R, X-linked recessive; A-R, autosomal recessive; A-D, autosomal dominant.
‡In view of recent data on this subject,[9] these figures are questionable.

ness of only one color. The monochromat has either a marked deficiency of normal cones (rod monochromat) or, more rarely, a transmission defect from the retina to the cerebral cortex (cone monochromat).

In addition, there are subjects with hypothesized minor color vision defects on the basis of slightly abnormal performance only on the anomaloscope.[1,2] (See p. 151.) In this group are subjects with only a wider than normal equation,* those who, after prolonged examinations, have wider than normal equations (color asthenopes), and those with a "shifted" equation just outside of the range of two standard deviations of the mean (color deviants). More data are necessary to define the color vision of individuals who have been included in these groups by some workers.

INCIDENCE AND INHERITANCE

The frequency of color blindness varies from about 1% to 13% of the male population, depending on the area of the world.[3-6] Post[7] analyzed frequency data and concluded that the incidence is highest in areas longest removed from food-gathering cultures. He attributes this remarkable difference to a "relaxation of natural selection" against a trait that was severely disadvantageous in hunting and food gathering cultures.

The incidence of color vision defects in American and European populations are summarized in Table 2. About 8% of all males and 0.5% of all females are color-blind. Deuteranomaly is the most common defect and protanomaly, deuteranopia, and protanopia, all of about equal incidence, are next in frequency. Rare color abnormalities include tritan defects, rod monochromatism, and cone monochromatism. Tetartanopia, a defect of questionable existence,[8] will not be considered in this discussion. Tritanopia is extremely rare and may actually be a manifestation of an hereditary optic nerve disease.[9]

---

*The meaning of an "equation" on the anomaloscope is discussed on p. 145.

Table 3. Color vision inheritance in females

| Genotype | | | | |
| Protan locus | | Deutan locus | | |
X_1	X_2	X_1	X_2	Phenotype
PA*	N	N	N	N
P	N	N	N	N
N	N	DA	N	N
N	N	D	N	N
PA	N	DA	N	N
PA	N	D	N	N
P	N	DA	N	N
P	N	D	N	N
PA	PA	N	N	PA
P	PA	N	N	PA
P	P	N	N	P
N	N	DA	DA	DA
N	N	D	DA	DA
N	N	D	D	D
PA	PA	DA	N	PA
PA	PA	DA	DA	Mixed

*PA, Protanomaly; P, protanopia; N, normal; DA, deuteranomaly; and D, deuteranopia. N is dominant to PA, P, DA, and D. PA is dominant to P. DA is dominant to D.

The most common types of color defects are inherited as X-linked recessive traits. Since the male has only one X chromosome, he will always manifest a color defect if he is carrying an abnormal gene. On the other hand, the female with two X chromosomes will usually not show the typical color defect unless she is carrying an abnormal gene on each chromosome for that defect. Exceptions to this rule will be considered later in this chapter.

There are now enough pedigrees to conclusively support the notion of two separate genetic loci for deutan and protan genes.[1,2,10-12] Supposedly, there are two series of multiple alleles, each of which has its own normal gene, its locus on the X chromosome, and its order of dominance.* Normal genes are dominant to protan and deutan genes. Mild defects are dominant to severe defects (for example, protanomaly is dominant to protanopia). There is no evidence, though, that any gene of the protan series is dominant or recessive to any gene of the deutan series. Thus, a male carrying genes of both series should show effects of each. However, a female carrying only one gene of each series may have normal color vision (Table 3). This latter fact is particularly against the one-locus hypothesis. The inheritance of the rarer color defects, shown in Table 2, will be considered in more detail when discussing these conditions.

---

*For example, protanopia, protanomaly, and possibly extreme protanomaly are the series of abnormal genes at one locus.

CLINICAL EVALUATION OF DEFECTIVE COLOR VISION

In defective color vision the three attributes of color sensation—brightness, hue, and saturation—are affected to a varying degree. Measurements of luminosity function, hue discrimination, and saturation discrimination, discussed in Chapter 5, are not usual clinical procedures. However, changes in these attributes enable a clearer understanding of each color defect and will be considered when discussing individual color defects.

The usual tests used clinically in evaluating color vision provide data that may be dependent on more than one attribute. Sometimes the relative importance of each attribute in a test is not clear. However, these tests are useful, to varying degrees, in answering the following questions: (1) Is the individual color defective or not? (2) What is the precise nature of the defect? (3) Is the defect acquired or congenital? (4) How does the defect incapacitate the individual? (5) Can an individual, whether or not he has a color defect, qualify for a vocation involving certain color judgments?

Sorting tests

The classical example of this type of test, the Holmgren wool test,[13] was produced in 1874 following a series of Swedish railroad accidents attributed to color blindness. This test involves the sorting of chromatic wool samples into three different groups in relation to three larger standard wool samples. The three standard test skeins are a very pale green, a light purple or pink, and a full red. The examiner selects a standard test skein and the examinee sorts out eight or ten of the smaller skeins having nearly the same color. The procedure is repeated with the other two standard test skeins in turn.

The Holmgren wool test suffers from lack of standardization, detects only about half of the color defectives examined, fails a number of "overanxious" normals, and permits easy practice improvement. Its main use is in the selection of fabric inspectors. Its only other possible use would be to test infants. The Montessori educational movement has shown that the matching and grouping of dyed skeins of wool is an activity that develops quite spontaneously during the play of children.

Pseudoisochromatic plates

The first series of pseudoisochromatic plates was published by Stilling in 1878.[14] Since then there have been many modifications of this original series and many other types of plates that have been published from several countries. In general, pseudoisochromatic plates are most useful for screening color defective from normal persons. Most of the data on incidence of color deficiency has been derived completely or in part from testing with plates.

Color defective persons confuse test symbols or numbers in pseudoisochromatic plates with the background. In most plates the colors of the test symbols and of the background are of such saturation, hue, and brightness that they are regularly confused by either the deutan or protan or both. However, in one series, the American Optical Company's Hardy-Rand-Rittler (H-R-R) plates, test symbol colors are close to the neutral points of deutans or protans and are thus confused to a varying degree with a gray background.

The most widely used set of pseudoisochromatic plates in the world at the present time is probably the Ishihara series. In comparative studies these plates usually prove to be as good or better than most other pseudoisochromatic series for screening purposes. These plates have been published in several editions since 1917. The most recent edition, published in 1962, consists of the sixteen best plates from previous editions. In general, this test consists of some plates in which the normal person sees one number and the color deficient another, some in which the numbers are read only by the normal subject, some in which the numbers are read only by the color deficient subject, and some in which a path has to be traced. The larger editions contain plates of questionable value for distinguishing between protan and deutan defects. The background and test dots on each plate are of varying size and varying hue. The test dots form either Arabic numerals or a multicurved continuous line. One criticism of the Ishihara plates is that some color defectives may pass as normals if a cut-off of three errors is used.[15] A cut-off of two missed plates should detect most color defectives but it is likely that too many normals will be misclassified.[16] Our suggestion is to use more than one pseudoisochromatic series for screening (we also use the American Optical Company's H-R-R plates).

Another popular test is the second edition of the H-R-R plates published in 1957. It consists of four demonstration, six screening, and fourteen diagnostic plates that test for both blue-yellow and red-green defects and also attempt to grade the severity of either defect. All subjects, regardless of the severity of their color defect, should identify the symbols on the four demonstration plates. On each plate there are circular dots of varying size. The background dots are neutral gray and the test dots are colored to form a symbol (a circle, a triangle, or a cross) placed in one or two quadrants of each plate. The dominant wavelengths of the test dots approximate the spectral and nonspectral neutral points of deutans and protans. Colors of low saturation are used as screening plates and three higher saturations are used for the diagnostic plates. The screening series should be repeated twice, since some normals missing one or two plates on the first trial will score correctly on the second trial.

The major criticism of this test is the misclassification of some normals as color defectives.*[15,17,18] However, there are several advantages that make this test quite useful in conjunction with another screening test such as the Ishihara:

1. It has blue-yellow plates, which are not found in most of the other pseudoisochromatic series.
2. The symbols are easy to teach to young children, illiterates, or those trained in other languages with different style numbers (for example, Arabic or Chinese), and therefore the test can be used in most subjects.
3. It is more accurate than most other pseudoisochromatic plates in classifying a defect as protan or deutan.[17,19]

The Rabkin plates are also good for this latter purpose.[19,20] However, no pseu-

---

*Occasionally color defectives are classified as normal.

doisochromatic plates are completely reliable in classifying red-green defects. We have tested color defectives in whom gross errors in classification were made with the H-R-R plates. Only the anomaloscope can be relied upon for the precise diagnosis of a red-green defect.

Other pseudoisochromatic plates that have received acclaim as screening plates include the Dvorine series,[14,19,21-23] published since 1944; the Russian Rabkin series,[19,23] published since 1939; and the Bostrom-Kugelberg series,[24] adopted as the official color test by the Royal Medical Board in Sweden. The Tokyo Medical College series attempts to classify and grade color defects as the H-R-R series does, but a critical analysis has shown it to be useful only as a screening test.[25] It also has plates to detect blue-yellow defects.

Farnsworth's hue discrimination tests[26-28]

Farnsworth devised two tests from paper chips selected from the Munsell Atlas of Colors differing in hue but having approximately the same saturation and brightness for normal subjects. In both tests the paper chips are mounted in black Bakelite caps and a complete color circle of hues is formed with approxi-

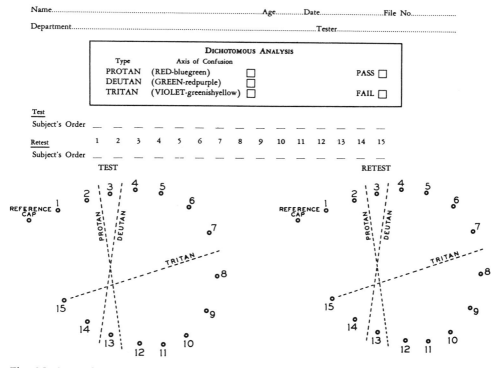

Fig. 6-1. Score sheet for the Farnsworth D-15 panel test, manufactured by the Psychological Corporation, New York City. The dotted lines show characteristic confusion axes for deutan, protan, and tritan defects. For example, an individual with a tritan type of defect would confuse caps 8 and 15 and therefore place cap 15 after cap 7.

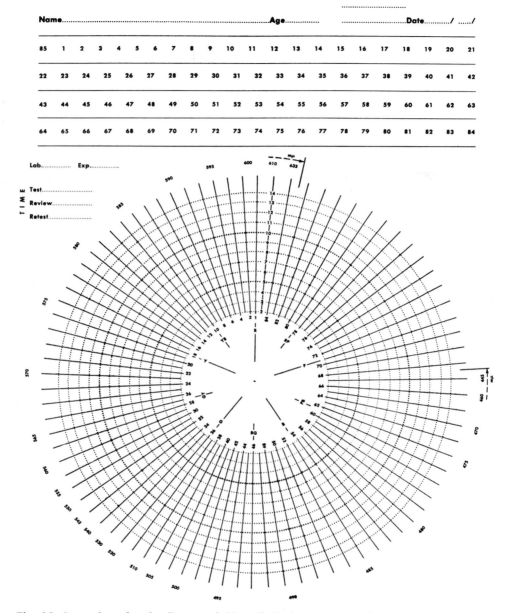

Fig. 6-2. Score sheet for the Farnsworth-Munsell 100-hue test manufactured by the Munsell Color Company, Inc., Baltimore. A polar coordinate diagram is shown with the circumference representing the eighty-five different caps and the radius representing the total number of errors for each removable cap. The score for a particular cap is calculated by subtracting the difference between the number of this cap and that of each adjacent cap and adding up these two differences. If an individual makes no errors, then the score for each cap should be 2 and the score would be plotted on the closest circle to the center. For example, considering cap 2, if it were in proper sequence it would be preceded by cap 1 and be followed by cap 3. The difference between cap 2 and cap 1 is one and similarly one for the difference between caps 3 and 2. Each succeeding circle is an increase in error score of 1.

mately equally discriminable hue steps between samples. The hue steps are much larger in the Farnsworth Dichotomous (D-15) test with sixteen paper chips than in the Farnsworth-Munsell 100-hue test, with eighty-five paper chips.

The Farnsworth D-15 test was designed to distinguish more severe color defectives from mild color defectives and normals. Thus there is a lower incidence of color blindness with this test than with pseudoisochromatic plates (5% compared to 8%). The test consists of a blue-violet chip fixed in position and fifteen other chips presented in random array. The subject attempts to arrange the caps in order starting with the chip closest to the reference cap. Dichromats and sufficiently affected anomalous trichromats will make two or more errors. From the axis of confusion, easily determined from the cleverly designed score sheet (Fig. 6-1), the defect is classified as either protan, deutan, or tritan. According to some workers[29] there are even characteristic axes for tetartanopia and total color blindness on this test.

The Farnsworth-Munsell 100-hue test was designed to separate persons with normal color vision into classes of superior, average, and low color discrimination and to measure zones of color confusion in color-defective persons. The

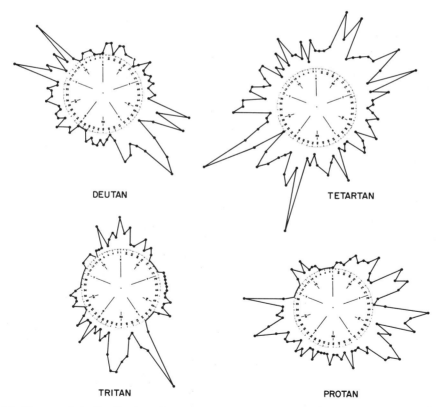

DEUTAN

TETARTAN

TRITAN

PROTAN

Fig. 6-3. Characteristic distribution of errors on the Farnsworth-Munsell 100-hue test for deutan, tetartan, tritan, and protan individuals.

eighty-five paper disks of this test are mounted in ninety-three caps divided into four boxes. Each box samples about one-fourth of the color circle and consists of twenty-one or twenty-two removable caps and two fixed pilot caps, one at each end of a case panel. The second pilot cap of one box is the same as the first of another box. The boxes and caps within are presented in random order. The subject arranges the removable caps in hue sequence between the two fixed end caps of each box. Scoring evaluates both the total errors and regions of greatest error concentration. The data are plotted on a polar coordinate diagram, with the circumference representing the eighty-five different caps and the radius representing the total number of errors for each removable cap (Fig. 6-2). Characteristic patterns (Fig. 6-3) readily identify the subject as deutan, protan, tritan or as having poor color discrimination with no particular pattern. The age of the subject must also be considered since normal older subjects (particularly beyond the age of 39) make more errors than younger subjects.[30,31] A few mild color defectives with good hue discrimination will be missed with this test; therefore, it is not recommended as a screening procedure.

Inter-Society Color Council color aptitude test

This test was developed to provide quantitative measures of color aptitude to be used in evaluating the suitability of workers for color-matching tasks and color-sorting operations.[32,87] An attempt is made to match fifty loose color samples to a panel of fifty fixed color samples. Color differences are small so that the normal may make many errors. On the other hand, some color defectives may perform adequately, for various reasons, so that this test cannot be used for screening or classification. Degree of color aptitude is indicated by the overall score on the test. The test can also be scored analytically with respect to performance in red, yellow, green, and blue areas. More control data are needed for this test.

Sloan achromatopsia test

The Sloan test is a good screening test for total color blindness. It uses six standard Munsell colors of high saturation covering the entire range of hues. Comparison of each color is made with a graduated series of seventeen grays. Only the achromat makes a match with the six saturated Munsell colors shown. Data on matches from nineteen patients with congenital total color blindness are used for comparison purposes.[33]

Illumination for tests

It should be emphasized that for all tests discussed so far, where pigments are used, the preferred illumination is that under which the test was standardized. In general the light from a Macbeth easel lamp, providing a white light of color temperature 6,740° K, is satisfactory. This light is equivalent to CIE Illuminant C source, which is considered representative of average daylight.[8] It is our experience and that of others[34,35] that results are most consistent when testing is done under the Macbeth easel lamp. Results obtained in fluorescent or incandescent backgrounds are not considered reliable in our experience, although one worker claims he gets consistent results on the Ishihara plates with a background of fluorescent lighting.[36]

Anomaloscope

A normal subject can match yellow in both color and brightness with a proper mixture of red and green. This match is frequently called the Rayleigh "equation" after Lord Rayleigh,[37] who discovered its usefulness in differentiating red-green color-blind individuals from normals.

The anomaloscope is an instrument designed to measure the Rayleigh equation. It is the only instrument by which the exact diagnosis of red-green color vision defects can be made. Several anomaloscopes have been designed, but the Nagel anomaloscope, named after the original designer, is the most widely used one. The instrument uses narrow band spectral lights from a prism and is in essence a combination of a spectroscope and a comparison polarimeter. The subject views a bipartite circular filed that is divided into a yellow half of variable luminance and a half with a variable red-green mixture of fixed luminance. Usually the examiner sets various red-green mixtures and the subject attempts to make brightness and, when possible, color matches by varying the yellow half of the field (fixed matches). Initially the subject may be allowed to manipulate both halves of the circular field (free matches), but these are usually less accurate than fixed matches. The examiner selects red-green mixtures to determine the range of matches satisfying color and brightness equality (Rayleigh equation) and to obtain brightness values and color identification at points over the entire range of the instrument. Some of the problems encountered when testing with this instrument have been summarized.[38] The characteristic findings for the various color defects will be described in the discussion of these defects.

Lantern tests

The lantern tests were designed primarily for occupation where the recognition of colored signals is the main or only discrimination involved. These tests are practical for screening tests for these occupations but are useless for diagnosing type or degree of color defect. The examinee is required to name colored lights presented at different luminance levels and at different visual angles (simulating distant signal lights). The U. S. Air Force uses the Sloan color-threshold test[39] and a popular test in the U. S. Navy is the Farnsworth New London Navy Lantern.[8] The lantern test presents paired rather than single colored signals. The luminance contrast between the paired test colors are chosen to eliminate cues from common brightness-hue relationships.

Screening for various occupations

One quickly learns that the presence of a color defect may not be a contraindication to a particular job. In fact, some color-defective individuals may perform better than some normals. Therefore one *cannot* rely only on pseudo-isochromatic plates for job screening. This has been vividly demonstrated in a study comparing the colorimetric performance of 800 normals and 800 subjects classified as color defectives by the Ishihara plates.[40] The job performance of the color-blind group was close to normal and most of the errors made were minor and described as "near misses." However, it may be argued that screening with plates is desirable for certain individuals such as train drivers or aircraft pilots, where perfect color vision is essential. For example, a train driver passes a colored light only once, sees it for a relatively brief period, and if he has mistaken the color there is no possibility of correcting his error. "Near misses" cannot be accepted.

Obviously screening color tests simulating work conditions are useful, particularly when fairly close agreement between actual performance and test results has been demonstrated. The lantern tests are good for the transportation services or armed forces. The Holmgren wool test may be good for fabric inspectors.

One test of probable predictive value for many industries is the Farnsworth D-15 test.[28,41] Some subjects failing the Farnsworth lantern test will even pass this test.[41] In general three out of eight color defectives will pass the D-15 test. The number of errors made on the Farnsworth-Munsell 100-hue test is helpful in evaluating the performance of color defectives. Those color defectives with a precise narrow match on the Nagel anomaloscope, in our experience, make fewer errors on the Farnsworth-Munsell 100-hue test than those with wider equations. In one study[42] it was shown that the greater the number of errors on a lantern test, the wider the equation on the Nagel anomaloscope for congenital color defectives. Color defectives classified as a dichromat or an extreme anomaly by the anomaloscope (see p. 150) tend to perform poorly in most color vision tasks. It is the common protanomalous and deuteranomalous subjects that have a great variation in performance.

In certain industries very critical color judgments are required (for example, color coding in various electrical industries). Even some normal subjects may not have satisfactory color performance and therefore screening with color aptitude tests may be helpful. The Farnsworth-Munsell 100-hue test is useful for this purpose since it divides all subjects into three groups according to performance. An even more critical appraisal of color vision performance is given by the Inter-Society Council color aptitude test.

CONGENITAL COLOR VISION DEFECTS
Rod monochromatism (achromatopsia with amblyopia)

Complete form. Photophobia, nystagmus, and visual acuity of about 20/200 are typical findings. Nystagmus may decrease for near so that reading vision is frequently better than distance vision. Photophobia and nystagmus, noted in most younger color-blind persons, may diminish or disappear as they become older, particularly beyond the age of 15 years. Visual acuity does not change significantly with age. The pupils may appear to be dilated in intense illumination because of an abnormally slow response to light, but pupillary responses during dark adaptation are normal. The eyegrounds show no or only minimal changes, such as absence of the foveal reflex. Discrete macular changes are occasionally seen.[1,54] The inheritance is autosomal recessive.

Colors are perceived only as shades of gray. Consequently there is a history of

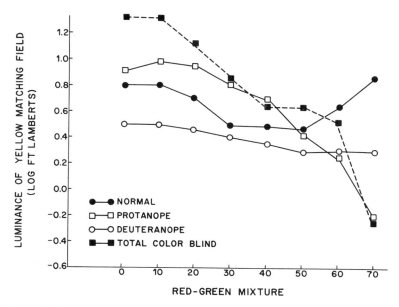

Fig. 6-4. Congenital color defects. Yellow brightness values on Nagel anomaloscope for various red-green mixtures for normal, protanope, deuteranope, and rod monochromat over range of instrument. On the X axis pure red is 70 and pure green is 0. All possible red-green mixtures are represented by intervening numbers. Luminance of yellow light is indicated on Y axis. Note that in the normal, red-green light is dimmest in region of match. In the deuteranope (and the deuteranomal as well) red-green mixtures are almost of equal brightness over the entire range of instrument. The protanope (and the protanomal) and the rod monochromat find red-green mixtures near the red end of the instrument to be very dim. In addition, the rod monochromat finds red-green mixtures near the green end of the instrument to be very bright. He may even turn the yellow light as bright as it will go and find that this is not enough for a brightness match.

difficulty in distinguishing colors; however, the symptoms may be minimized because of educational and environmental factors. Many color-blind persons learn to associate colors with objects and may skillfully make many color judgments by discerning differences in brightness. Of course, in test situations difference in brightness can be eliminated and these subjects can be easily identified.

Pronounced abnormalities are seen on all color vision tests. Most plates on any pseudoisochromatic series are missed. A color match is made over the entire range of the anomaloscope, but brightness matches are usually made only at the red end of the instrument (Fig. 6-4). The latter finding is unique for total color blindness. Large errors are made over the entire Farnsworth-Munsell 100-hue test with no definite axis. According to Verriest and co-workers,[29] a typical axis, though, is found on the Farnsworth dichotomous test. On the Sloan achromatopsia cards the subject is able to make perfect matches to all six hues. The luminosity curve is of the scotopic type at all illuminations.

Visual fields may be normal or slightly constricted, particularly to colors, and sometimes a central scotoma can be demonstrated; however, nystagmus may make this testing difficult. The ERG shows unique diagnostic findings that are an absence or marked diminution of the single-flash photopic response and of the first portion of a scotopic orange-red response and a low flicker fusion frequency.[43]

Incomplete forms. The findings for incomplete forms are the same as in the complete form but less in degree. Photophobia and nystagmus may be absent and visual acuity less impaired. Sloan and Newhall[44] even reported one patient with acuity of 20/40. The chromatic defect is usually incomplete for certain colors and may vary with the size of the field and the level of luminance. Photopic luminosity function is usually of the scotopic type at lower photopic luminance levels, but in some patients it becomes photopic or mixed at higher luminances.[45-48] Hue discrimination may resemble that of a dichromat and sometimes even that of an anomalous trichromat. The ERG shows the same diagnostic changes as in the complete form, but frequently to a lesser degree.

The various forms of total color blindness probably reflect the total number and type of abnormal or missing cones. Probably, though, some functioning cones are always present.

Histological studies of this disorder all showed the presence of some anatomically normal cones.[49-51] Psychophysical tests show evidence of cone activity in "complete" forms of total color blindness.[52-54] It is obvious that the distinction between "complete" and "incomplete" forms is frequently only a matter of degree and depends on the parameter considered. Support for the hypothesis that both types are usually only modifications of one genotype comes from the finding of both complete and incomplete forms in members of three families.[1]

There appear to be, on the other hand, two unique types of incomplete rod monochromatism. In one blue cones are minimally or not involved. Since these cones probably represent only a small portion of all retinal cones, the ERG is just as abnormal as in the typical complete form.[55,56] These patients have a photopic or mixed luminosity curve at high photopic intensities and a scotopic type at low photopic intensities.[46,47] There is also evidence of blue cone function on certain psychophysical tests. Since the inheritance is sex-linked recessive, only males have this condition; however, minor abnormalities have been reported in female carriers.[57-59]

The other type of incomplete rod monochromatism appears to involve mainly macular cones. The diagnostic finding in this condition is close to normal flicker frequency on the ERG with markedly abnormal single flash photopic and scotopic red responses. We have studied four such patients from one family and the inheritance is definitely autosomal recessive.[43] Other than the unique ERG these patients were similar to others with incomplete rod monochromatism. Incomplete achromats with normal or close to normal fusion frequencies have been also reported by Elenius and Zwei[60] (two cases) and Pabst and Echte[61] (two cases). The existence of this condition was definitely confirmed by the histological study of an achromatic eye showing abnormal cones only in the fovea.[49]

Cone monochromatism (achromatopsia without amblyopia)

Cone monochromatism is a very rare form of total color blindness characterized by minimal or no evidence of cone abnormality. There is normal visual acuity, no nystagmus or photophobia, normal eyegrounds, and usually normal visual fields. The position of the luminosity maximum may be normal or shifted to the short or long wavelength end of the spectrum, and there may be a shortening of one or both ends of the luminosity curve. Frequently these subjects have some degree of color vision, depending on the saturation of the colors used, the luminance level, and the size of the test field.[44,62-64] The inheritance is uncertain.

It is possible that this is a mixed group of subjects having combination receptor defects, postreceptoral defects, or both. Evidence favoring a combination receptor defect is the finding of independent protan, deutan, and tritan defects in relatives of these subjects.[62-64] However, if cone monochromatism were caused by the combination of an acquired blue-yellow defect together with a congenital red-green defect, a much higher incidence than about one case in 100 million population[64] should be detected, since both acquired blue-yellow defects and congenital double protan-deutan defects are not too uncommon. Also, the theory of combination defects does not explain the relation of the chromatic defect to the level of luminance in some cases,[62,63] the presence of a differential accommodative response to colors,[65] and the normal ERG in three patients[66-68] (a protan defect produces an ERG abnormality[43]). These data support the concept of a postreceptoral defect.

Dichromatism

Of the three types described only two, protanopia and deuteranopia, occur to a significant degree (Table 2). Tritanopia is extremely rare and may actually be a manifestation of a hereditary optic nerve disease.[9] Protanopia and deuteranopia are sex-linked recessive traits whereas tritanopia is an autosomal dominant defect.

The dichromat can match all the colors he experiences with appropriate mixtures of two colors. The number of colors remaining chromatic varies with the type of dichromatism, but in all these are interpreted as various saturations of only two hues. These hues are blue and yellow for the protanope and deuteranope and red and green for the tritanope. For each, the saturation decreases to zero at two points in the hue circle called neutral points. These are: (1) 495 nm and its complementary for the protanope, (2) 500 nm and its complementary for the deuteranope, and (3) 572 nm and its complementary for the tritanope. The colors confused by dichromats are best illustrated by the connecting lines on a chromaticity diagram, discussed in Chapter 5. Protanopes have confusion zones that converge toward the red end of the spectrum so that they tend to make confusions among red, gray, and bluish blue-green. Deuteranopic confusion zones tend to run parallel to the red-green direction and thus the deuteranope makes confusions among purple, gray, and greenish blue-green. Tritanopic confusion zones converge toward the violet end of the spectrum, so that they tend to make confusions among yellow, gray, and bluish purple. Diagnosis of these conditions on the anomaloscope is based in part by the tendency of protanopes and deuteranopes to confuse red and green with yellow and the tritanope to confuse green and blue with cyan.*

---

*No commercially available anomaloscope produces this match.

The protanope usually recognizes his color defect because of blindness at the far red end of the visible spectrum so that no light stimuli beyond 680 nm are seen. The brightest colors he sees under photopic conditions are near 540 nm (instead of near 560 nm as in the normal person). On the other hand, the deuteranope has a near normal relative luminosity function and thus frequently is unaware of his defect. It is questionable whether the relative luminosity loss in the blue and green spectral regions that some deuteranopes may show[69] produces symptoms.

The pseudoisochromatic plates are inadequate for distinguishing the protanope from the deuteranope or the dichromat from the anomalous trichromat. The Farnsworth-Munsell 100-hue test and the Farnsworth dichotomous test distinguish the protan from the deutan subject but do not classify the defect as dichromatic or trichromatic. Only the anomaloscope enables a clear-cut diagnosis. Both dichromats can make color and brightness matches over most of the range of the anomaloscope by simply changing tht brightness of the yellow half of the bipartite field (Fig. 6-5). However, the protanope uses a very dim yellow light near the red end of the instrument (he frequently cannot make the yellow light dark enough), while the deuteranope uses about the same yellow brightness in all matches (Fig. 6-4). Anomaloscope findings in anomalous trichromats will be considered in the next section.

The tritanope may be abnormal at the blue end of the spectrum but existent data show considerable variability. If he has such an abnormality, he will be aware of a color defect. The missing of only blue-yellow plates on the H-R-R pseudoisochromatic series and the finding in both eyes of a tritan axis on either the Farnsworth-Munsell 100-hue test or Farnsworth dichotomous test, without

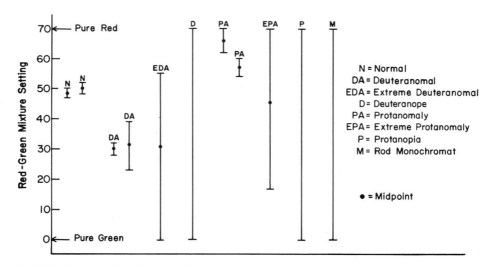

Fig. 6-5. Position of Rayleigh match (equation) on Nagel anomaloscope. Midpoints are shown for normal and the anomalous trichromats. On the Y axis all possible red-green mixtures are represented with pure red as 70 and pure green as 0.

previous or present retinal or optic nerve disease, suggests this diagnosis (or that of tritanomaly). There are no commercial anomaloscopes available for distinguishing the dichromat from the trichromat with a tritan defect, although some workers have designed their own instrumentation.[86] The finding of a neutral point between 579 to 585 nm identified a subject as a tritanope. As indicated, tritan abnormalities are inherited as autosomal dominant traits.[70] The gene has a marked variability of expression, so that tritanopia and tritanomaly may be found in the same family.[71] This is in contrast to red-green dichromatic and trichromatic defects, which usually do not appear in the same family unless a phenotypically anomalous female is carrying one gene for the anomaly and one also for a dichromacy (see discussion on p. 137). All of the findings described for congenital tritan defects can be seen in patients with hereditary dominant optic atrophy.[9]

Anomalous trichromatism

Probably most protanomalous trichromats are aware of a color defect because of blindness at the red end of the spectrum. In fact, the loss at the red end of the spectrum in protanomals may be as severe as that noted in the protanope. Deuteranomals frequently are unaware of their color problem.

In contrast to dichromats, anomalous trichromats have no neutral points under favorable conditions of lighting with large stimuli. However, even with trichromatic color vision these subjects distinguish only about five to twenty-five hues compared to over 150 that the normal person identifies. Similar to the normal, they frequently have only a relatively narrow region of brightness and color match on the anomaloscope. However, the deuteranomal requires at least four times more green than the normal and the protanomal at least one and a half times more red than normal in their Rayleigh equations. As a consequence, the position of the brightness and color match gives the diagnosis (Figs. 6-4 and 6-5). Sometimes the protanomal has a borderline equation, but he can be identified by the very dim yellow light he uses to match brightness at the red end of the instrument. Another anomaloscopic finding, called the "heightened contrast" phenomenon, distinguishes the protanomal from the normal subject. Yellow next to green light is often identified as a red light by the protan, whereas it is seen as yellow by the normal. The tritanomal theoretically requires more than a normal amount of blue in blue-green mixture to match a given blue-green, but at present no clinical instrument is available for studying this equation.

Franceschetti[72] has also proposed the existence of two other distinct forms of red-green anomaly that he calls extreme protanomaly and extreme deuteranomaly. These subjects are detected by anomaloscopic examination. The extreme protanomal will match the red-green mixture to yellow in color and brightness except when pure and close to pure green is used; the extreme deuteranomal does the same except when pure red or close to pure red is used (Fig. 6-5). These subjects are distinguished from dichromats by the absence of a neutral point[73] as well as by anomaloscopic findings.

Waardenburg and his colleagues[1] question whether extreme and regular anomalies are distinct entities. He points out that the two may be seen in the same family and that factors of adaptation and "exhaustion" may cause marked widening of the Rayleigh equation in some anomals.

Status of the female carrier of red-green defects

A female with two defective genes (a homozygote) will be color-blind, like the male with one defective gene (Table 3). However, color defects have also been noted in females with only one defective gene (a heterozygote). A few of these females have only one X chromosome[74] (Turner's syndrome); however, most have two.

Females heterozygous for either protan or deutan genes have been reported to show a variety of mild color vision abnormalities.[1,75-77] The two most frequently reported abnormalities are: (1) a mild to moderately severe defect on the anomaloscope in either the protan or deutan defect carrier,[73,75] and (2) a moderate to severe decrease in sensitivity to red light in the protan defect carriers.[88,89] A hue discrimination defect was also demonstrated in protan carriers with the Farnsworth-Munsell 100-hue test.[30] There is no completely satisfactory explanation for females with one X chromosome who show color vision abnormalities, which are usually mild but on occasion as severe as that found in the male. A recent theory that attempts to explain the status of the female carrier of X-linked defects is the Lyon hypothesis.[59]

Acquired color vision defects

Acquired color vision defects are caused by diseases of the macula, optic nerve, or occipital cortex or by cataracts. Certain findings aid in distinguishing acquired and congenital color vision defects.
  1. Congenital defects are likely to be bilateral and symmetrical. An acquired defect may be of greater degree in one eye than the other, may be unilateral, or may occasionally even be confined to various parts of the visual field of one eye. For example, a patient with a spotty macular lesion may give variable results on the anomaloscope by slight changes in direction of gaze.
  2. Acquired defects frequently involve blue-yellow as well as red-green discriminations, whereas congenital defects usually involve only the latter.
  3. Acquired color defects are usually associated with other evidence of abnormal retinal function (for example, abnormal visual acuity or visual fields). Congenital color defects, except for total color blindness, are essentially associated with normal retinal function.
  4. Congenital defects are said to be less dependent on testing conditions. Size, brightness, and saturation of objects are more likely to affect color discrimination of an acquired defect.
  5. A more rapid fatiguing develops for all colors on color vision testing with acquired color vision defects.[81]
  6. Subjects with acquired defects name the color of objects as they see them, whereas patients with congenital defects or long-established acquired defects are markedly affected by psychological considerations as to what the color of an object should be.[81] Other differences have also been cited.[1,81]

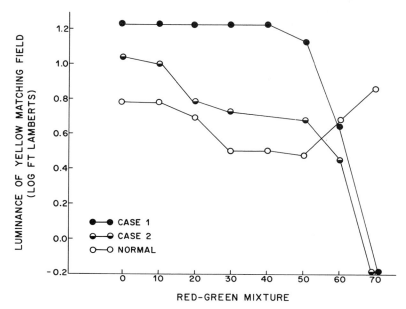

Fig. 6-6. Yellow brightness values on Nagel anomaloscope for various red-green mixtures over range of instrument for two patients with cone degenerations. Note that the yellow light is turned very bright at the green end of the instrument and very dim at the red end of the instrument, similar to what is seen in the totally color blind individual (see Fig. 6-4).

In the past, it has been stated that retinal disease is more likely to be characterized by blue-yellow defects and optic nerve disease by red-green defects. This distinction is meaningless, since a wide variety of color vision disturbances are found in such diseases.* Data from two tests, the Nagel anomaloscope and the Farnsworth-Munsell 100-hue test, enable the division of acquired defects into five distinct groups:

1. Patients with cone dystrophies are frequently characterized initially by a deutan axis on the 100-hue test and a very wide Rayleigh equation on the anomaloscope. In many of these patients pure green on the anomaloscope appears very bright and pure red very dim (Fig. 6-6). Their color vision data may be similar to that found in congenital total color blindness. Indeed, similar ERG data may also be found in the two conditions.[83,91]

2. Patients with hereditary dominant optic atrophy are initially characterized by a tritan axis on the 100-hue test and usually a normal performance on the anomaloscope.

3. Patients with macular diseases, other than a cone degeneration, are characterized usually by a wider than normal Rayleigh equation on the anomaloscope, requiring more red than normal in this equation, and having

---

*See references 1, 31, 78 to 82, and 90.

a tritan axis on the 100-hue test. The anomaloscope usually shows an abnormality before the 100-hue test.

4. Patients with optic nerve diseases, other than hereditary dominant optic atrophy and glaucoma, are usually characterized initially by a deutan axis on the 100-hue test and a wider than normal Rayleigh equation on the anomaloscope. These patients also required more green than normal in their Rayleigh equation. Occasionally, a patient in this category will show a tritan axis on the 100-hue test.

5. Patients with glaucoma, particularly with optic nerve damage, may show similar findings to those with most macular diseases. However, an abnormality is seen with the 100-hue test before it is detected on the anomaloscope, in contrast to what is found in patients with macular disease.

It should be emphasized that in advanced macular or optic nerve disease, particularly with vision worse than 20/200, these distinctions break down.

In general, the brightness of pure red and green lights on the anomaloscope is normal in most patients with acquired retinal or optic nerve diseases. Notable exceptions are most patients with cone degenerations and a few with optic nerve disease who find predominately green lights to be brighter than normal and predominately red lights to be dimmer than normal. A few patients with optic nerve disease find predominately red lights to be brighter than normal and predominately green lights to be dimmer than normal.

As a rule, patients with amblyopia ex anopsia and congenital retinal abnormalities, such as albinism and congenital nightblindness with abnormal vision, have only mild color vision abnormalities. On the other hand, patients with cone degenerations, chloroquine retinopathy, toxic amblyopia, and sometimes central serous choroidopathy are characterized by prominent color vision disturbances, even with a minimal visual acuity abnormality.

No specific color vision abnormalities characterize disease of the occipital cortex,[84,85] but not enough data are available.

REFERENCES

1. Waardenburg, P. J., Franceschetti, A., and Klein, D.: Genetics and ophthalmology, vol. 2, Springfield, Ill., 1963, Charles C Thomas, Publisher, pp. 1422-1566.
2. Pickford, R. W.: The genetics of colour blindness, Brit. J. Physiol. Optics 21:39, 1964.
3. Pickford, R. W.: Individual differences in colour vision, London, 1951, Routledge and Kegan Paul Ltd.
4. Dutta, P. C.: A review of the inherited defective colour-vision variability and selection relaxation among the Indians, Acta Genet. 16:327, 1966.
5. Roberts, D. F.: Red/green color blindness in the Niger Delta, Eugen. Quart. 14:7, 1967.
6. Salzano, F. M.: Color blindness among Indians from Santa Catarma, Brazil, Acta Genet. 14:219, 1964.
7. Post, R. H.: Population differences in red and green color-vision deficiency, Eugen. Quart. 9:131, 1962.
8. Committee on Colorimetry, Optical Society of America: The science of color, New York, 1953, Thomas Y. Crowell Co.
9. Krill, A. E., Smith, V. C., and Pokorny, J.: Further studies supporting the identity of congenital tritanopia and hereditary atrophy, Invest. Ophthal. 10:182, 1971.
10. Dreyer, V., and Goldschmidt, E.: The offspring of two color blind parents, Acta Genet. 15:97, 1965.

11. Vanderdonck, R., and Verriest, G.: Femme protanomale et héterozygote mixte ayant deux fils deuteranopes, un fils protanomal et deux fils normaux, Biotypologie **21**:110, 1960.
12. Siniscalco, M., and Fillippi, G.: Recombination between protan and deutan genes; data on their relative positions in respect of the GGPD locus, Nature **204**:1062, 1964.
13. Collins, M.: Color-blindness, New York, 1925, Harcourt, Brace, Jovanovich.
14. Linksz, A.: An essay on color vision and clinical color-vision tests, New York, 1964, Grune and Stratton, Inc.
15. Sloan, L. L., and Habel, A.: Tests for color deficiency based on the pseudo-isochromatic principle: a comparative study of several new tests, Arch. Ophthal. (Chicago) **55**:229, 1956.
16. Krill, A. E., Bowman, J. E., and Schneiderman, A.: An investigation of so-called X-linked errors on the Ishihara plates, Ann. Hum. Genet. **29**:253, 1966.
17. Crone, R. A.: Quantitative diagnosis of defective color vision: a comparative evaluation of the Ishihara test, the Farnsworth dichotomous test, and the Hardy Rand Rittler polychromatic plates, Amer. J. Ophthal. **51**:298, 1961.
18. Walls, G.: How good is the H-R-R test for color blindness? Amer. J. Optom. **36**:169, 1959.
19. Frey, R. G.: Zur Differentialdiagnose der angeborenen Farbensinnstörungeun mit pseudo-isochromatischen Tafeln, Ophthalmologica **145**:34, 1963.
20. Hardy, L. H., Rand, R., and Rittler, M. C.: Test for the detection and analysis of color blindness. III: Rabkin test, J. Opt. Soc. Amer. **35**:481, 1945.
21. Crawford, A.: The Dvorine pseudo-isochromatic plates, Brit. J. Psychol. **46**:139, 1955.
22. Dvorine, I.: Quantitative classification of the color blind, J. Gen. Psychol. **68**:255, 1963.
23. Babel, J.: Diagnostic des dyschromatopsies congenitales et acquisés, Ophthalmologica **149**:277, 1965.
24. Bostrom, C. G., and Kugelberg, I.: Official color sense control in Sweden, Arch. Ophthal. (Chicago) **38**:378, 1947.
25. Sloan, L. L.: Evaluation of the Tokyo-Medical College color vision test, Amer. J. Ophthal. **52**:650, 1961.
26. Farnsworth, D.: The Farnsworth-Munsell 100 hue and dichotomous tests for color vision, J. Opt. Soc. Amer. **33**:568, 1943.
27. Pedriel, G.: Le test de Farnsworth 100 hue, Ann. Oculist. **195**:120, 1962.
28. Linksz, A.: Farnsworth dichotomous test, Amer. J. Ophthal. **62**:27, 1966.
29. Verriest, G., Buyssens, A., and Vanderdonck, R.: Etude quantitative de l'effet qu'éxércé sur les résultats de quelques tests de la discrimination chromatique une diminution non selective du niveau d'un éclairage, C. Rev. Opt. **42**:105, 1963.
30. Krill, A. E., and Schneiderman, A.: A hue discrimination defect in so-called normal carriers of color vision defects, Invest. Ophthal. **3**:445, 1964.
31. Verriest, G.: Further studies on acquired deficiency of color discrimination, J. Opt. Soc. Amer. **53**:185, 1963.
32. Collins, W. E., Casola, A. S., and Zegers, R. T.: The performance of color-blind subjects on the color aptitude test, J. Gen. Psychol. **64**:245, 1961.
33. Sloan, L. L.: Congenital achromatopsia: a report of 19 cases, J. Opt. Soc. Amer. **44**:117, 1954.
34. Schmidt, I.: Effect of illumination in testing color vision with pseudo-isochromatic plates, J. Opt. Soc. Amer. **42**:951, 1952.
35. Hardy, H. L.: Standard illuminants in relation to color testing procedures, Arch. Ophthal. (Chicago) **34**:278, 1945.
36. Katavisto, M.: Pseudo-isochromatic plates and artificial light, Acta Ophthal. **39**:377, 1961.
37. Rayleigh, Lord: Experiments on colour, Nature **25**:64, 1881.
38. Schmidt, I.: Some problems related to testing color vision with the Nagel anomaloscope, J. Opt. Soc. Amer. **45**:514, 1955.
39. Sloan, L. L.: A quantitative test for measuring degree of red-green color deficiency, Amer. J. Ophthal. **27**:941, 1944.
40. Fetter, M. C.: Colorimetric tests read by color-blind people, Amer. J. Med. Tech. **29**:349, 1963.
41. Farnsworth, D.: Testing for color deficiency in industry, Arch. Ind. Health **16**:100, 1957.
42. Cameron, G. R.: Rational approach to color vision testing, Aerospace Med. **38**:51, 1967.

43. Krill, A. E.: The electroretinogram in congenital color vision defects: the clinical value of electroretinography, ISCERG Symposium, 1966, Basel, 1968, S. Karger A. G.

44. Sloan, L. L., and Newhall, S. M.: Comparison of atypical and typical achromatopsia, Amer. J. Ophthal. **25**:945, 1942.

45. Jaeger, W.: Systematische Untersuchungen über inkomplette angeborene totale Farbenblind-heit, Graefe. Arch. Ophthal. **150**:509, 1950; Typen der inkompletten Achromatopsie, Ber Deutsch. Ophthal. Ges. **58**:44, 1953.

46. Blackwell, H., and Blackwell, O.: Rod and cone receptor mechanisms in typical and atypical congenital achromatopsia, Vis. Res. **1**:62, 1961.

47. Alpern, M., Lee, G. B., and Spivey, B. E.: Pi_1 monochromatism, Arch. Ophthal. (Chicago) **74**:334, 1965.

48. Siegel, I. M., and others: Analysis of photopic and scotopic function in an incomplete achromat, J. Opt. Soc. Amer. **56**:699, 1966.

49. Larsen, H., and Lauber, H.: Demonstration mikroskopischer: Praaparate von einem mono-chromatischen, Klin. Mbl. Augenheilk. **67**:301, 1921.

50. Harrison, R., Hoefnagel, D., and Hayward, J. N.: Congenital total color blindness: a clinico-pathological report, Arch. Ophthal. (Chicago) **64**:685, 1960.

51. Falls, H. F., Wolter, J. R., and Alpern, M.: Typical total monochromacy, Arch. Ophthal. (Chicago) **74**:610, 1965.

52. Walls, G., and Heath, G.: Typical total color blindness reinterpreted, Acta Ophthal. **32**:253, 1954.

53. Sloan, L. L.: The photopic retinal receptors of the typical achromat, Amer. J. Ophthal. **46**:81, 1958.

54. Alpern, M., Falls, H. F., and Lee, G. B.: The enigma of typical total monochromacy, Amer. J. Ophthal. **50**:996, 1960.

55. François, J., and Verriest, G.: Trois nouvelles observations d'achromatopsie congenitale atypique, Ann. Oculist. (Paris) **193**:123, 1960.

56. Spivey, B. E.: The X-linked recessive inheritance of atypical monochromatism, Arch. Oph-thal. (Chicago) **74**:327, 1965.

57. Krill, A. E.: A technique for evaluating photopic and scotopic flicker function with one light intensity, Docum. Ophthal. **18**:452, 1964.

58. Spivey, B. E., Pearlman, J. T., and Burian, H. M.: Electroretinographic findings (including flicker) in carriers of congenital X-linked achromatopsia, Docum. Ophthal. **18**:367, 1964.

59. Krill, A. E.: X-chromosomal-linked diseases affecting the eye: status of the heterozygote female, Trans. Amer. Ophthal. Soc. **67**:535, 1969.

60. Elenius, V., and Zwei, M.: Flicker electroretinography in six cases of total colour blindness, Acta Ophthal. **36**:19, 1958.

61. Pabst, W., and Echte, K.: Die Unterschiedsempfindlichkeitsschwelle bei Achromaten bestimmt mit hilf des Electroretinogramms, Acta Ophthal. **70** (Supp.):168, 1962.

62. Weale, R. A.: Cone monochromatism, J. Physiol. **121**:548, 1953.

63. Crone, R. A.: Combined forms of congenital color defects: a pedigree with atypical total color blindness, Brit. J. Ophthal. **40**:462, 1956.

64. Pitt, F. H. G.: Monochromatism, Nature **154**:466, 1944.

65. Fincham, E. F.: The effect of colour deficiency on the accommodation reflex, J. Physiol. **121**:570, 1953.

66. Blumgardt, E.: Un cas d'achromatopsie atypique, J. Physiol. (Paris) **47**:83, 1955.

67. Ikeda, H., and Ripps, H.: The electroretinogram of a cone monochromat, Arch. Ophthal. **75**:315, 1966.

68. Krill, A. E., and Schneiderman, A.: Retinal function studies, including the electroretino-gram, in an atypical monochromat. In Francois, J., editor: Clinical electroretinography, New York, 1966, Oxford Press, pp. 351-361.

69. Hsia, Y., and Graham, C. H.: Spectral luminosity curves for protanopic, deuteranopic, and normal subjects, Proc. Nat. Acad. Sci. **43**:1011, 1957.

70. Kalmus, H.: The familial distribution of congenital tritanopia with some remarks on some similar conditions, Ann. Hum. Genet. **20**:39, 1955.

71. Cole, B. L., Henry, G. H., and Nathan, J.: Phenotypical variation of tritanopia, Vis. Res. **6**: 301, 1966.

72. Franceschetti, A.: Die Bedeutung der Einstellungsbreite am Anomaloskop für die Diagnose der einzelnen Typen der Farbsinnstörungen, nebst Bemerkungen über ihren Vererbungsmodus, Schweiz. Med. Wschr. **58**:1273, 1928.

73. Walls, G., and Mathews, R.: New means of studying color blindness and normal foveal color vision, U. Calif. Pub. Psychol. **7**:1, 1952.

74. Walls, G. L.: Peculiar color blindness in peculiar people, Arch. Ophthal. (Chicago) **62**:13, 1959.

75. François, J.: Heredity in ophthalmology, St. Louis, 1961, The C. V. Mosby Co.

76. Adam, A.: Foveal red-green ratios of normals, colour-blinds, and heterogyzotes, Proc. Tel-Hashomer Hosp. **8**:2, 1968.

77. Crone, R. A.: Spectral sensitivity in color defective subjects and heterozygous carriers, Amer. J. Ophthal. **48**:231, 1959.

78. Verriest, G.: Les déficiences acquisés de la discrimination chromatique, Bull. Acad. Roy. Med. Belg. **4**:37, 1964.

79. Grutzner, P.: Über erworbene Farbensinnstörungen bei Sehnervenerkrankungen: V, Graefe. Arch. Ophthal. **169**:366, 1966.

80. Hong, S.: Types of acquired color vision defects, Arch. Ophthal. (Chicago) **58**:505, 1957.

81. Jaeger, W.: Defective color vision caused by eye disease, Trans. Ophthal. Soc. U.K. **76**:477, 1956.

82. Gibson, H. C., Smith, D. M., and Alpern, M.: Pi_5 specificity in digitoxin toxicity, Arch. Ophthal. (Chicago) **74**:154, 1965.

83. Goodman, G., Ripps, H., and Siegel, I. M.: Cone dysfunction syndromes, Arch. Ophthal. (Chicago) **70**:214, 1963.

84. L'Hermite, F., and others: Les troubles de la vision des couleurs dans les lesions postérieures du cerveau, Rev. Neurol. **121**:5, 1969.

85. Geschwund, G., and Fusillo, M.: Color-naming defects in association with alexia, Arch. Neurol. **15**:137, 1966.

86. Pickford, R. W., and Lakowsky, R.: The Pickford-Nicholson anomaloscope for testing and measuring colour sensitivity and colour-blindness, Brit. J. Physiol. Opt. **17**:131, 1960.

87. Dimmick, F. L.: A color aptitude test, 1940 experimental edition, J. Appl. Psychol. **30**:10, 1946.

88. Schmidt, I.: Ueber manifeste Heterozygotie bei Konduktorinnen für Farbensinnstörungen, Klin. Mbl. Augenheilk. **92**:456, 1934.

89. Krill, A. E., and Beutler, E.: Red-light thresholds in heterozygote carriers of protanopia: genetic implications, Science **149**:186, 1965.

90. Krill, A. E., and Fishman, G. A.: Acquired color vision defects, Trans. Amer. Acad. Ophthal. Otolaryng. **75**:1095, 1971.

91. Krill, A. E.: The electroretinographic and electrooculographic findings in patients with macular lesions, Trans. Amer. Acad. Ophthal. Otolaryng. **70**:1063, 1966.

APPENDIX

The following addresses may be of value for those interested in purchasing the following equipment:

Farnsworth D-15 Panel Test
  The Psychological Corporation
  304 East 45th Street
  New York, N. Y. 10017
Nagel Anomaloscope
  Alfred P. Poll
  40 West 55th Street
  New York, N. Y. 10019

Macbeth Easel Lamp or Farnsworth-Munsell
  100-Hue Test
  Munsell Color Company, Inc.
  2441 North Calvert Street
  Baltimore, Md. 21218

PART IV Special topics in
visual function

CHAPTER *7 Practical aspects of depth perception*

HERMANN M. BURIAN

Man's orientation in space in the third dimension is based on two sets of clues: binocular (stereoscopic) and monocular (nonstereoscopic) clues. When a person who has always enjoyed normal binocular vision acutely loses the vision of one eye, he will be annoyed by certain unexpected difficulties in functioning in space. He may have difficulties in pouring cream in his coffee cup and in the performance of other visuomanual tasks. These difficulties arise because of the sudden loss of the binocular (stereoscopic) clues to depth perception. In time the patient overcomes his handicap and may become almost as skillful as he was before he lost his eye, although fast-moving objects, such as a flying ball, may continue to give him trouble. He learns to rely more and more on monocular (nonstereoscopic) clues to depth perception, even in near vision, where he formerly relied almost entirely on binocular clues. A brief review of the two sets of clues is thus necessary as a background for the discussion of the practical aspects of depth perception.

STEREOPSIS[1]

Every visual sensation, whether produced by the adequate stimulus, light, or by an inadequate stimulus, such as blow or an electrical current, is always localized in a specific position in visual space. This is caused by the fact that each retinocortical element possesses an inherent spatial value. Any stimulus reaching a retinocortical element outside the foveola is localized in a specific visual direction, relative to the visual direction of the foveola; this direction is known as the *principal subjective visual direction.* This relationship is *quantitative,* depending on the position and distance of the retinocortical element with respect to the foveola, and *immutable* in that it is independent of changes in the position of the foveola. One may say that each retinocortical element transmits a specific *relative subjective visual direction.* It is this characteristic of the visual system that makes an orderly visual field possible.

Now, the organization of man's visual system is such that each retinocortical element in one eye has a partner in the other eye that has the identical relative subjective visual direction. This is true for the foveolas, which carry the *principal subjective common visual direction,* and for all other retinal elements within the field of binocular vision. All of them have a *common relative subjective visual direction,* quantitatively related to the principal common visual direction. Partners of this type are designated as *corresponding retinocortical elements.*

One object localized in *one* direction—for example, the fixation point—must necessarily be seen singly, even though it stimulates two spatially separated retinal elements, one in each eye. It is impossible to see doubly when corresponding elements are simultaneously stimulated. Single vision so produced is the basis of *sensory fusion.*

If an object is presented in such a fashion as not to stimulate corresponding retinocortical elements in the two eyes, it will stimulate elements having different relative subjective directions, so-called *noncorresponding* or *disparate elements.* If an object appears at the same time in two directions, this means that it must be seen in diplopia. Disparity is the basis of double vision. Well-known examples of this are the so-called physiological diplopia—that is, the doubling up of an object located nearer or farther than the fixation point—and the diplopia experienced by patients who have acutely acquired a paresis of an extraocular muscle.

The distribution of the directional values of the retinocortical elements is not strictly a geometrical one. It differs in the two eyes of the same person and, within narrow limits, from individual to individual. Their actual distribution must be determined by experiment. This is most readily done by having the observer fixate a vertical rod placed at a near vision distance in the midplane of his head (Fig. 7-1). The rod is seen through an aperture against a uniform background and the head is carefully adjusted. To each side of the fixated rod are a number of movable rods, seen in peripheral vision. To determine the distribution of corresponding retinocortical elements, a number of criteria may be em-

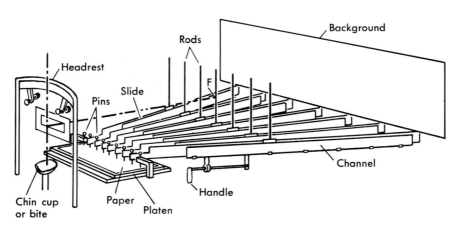

Fig. 7-1. Schematic drawing of horopter apparatus. The rods are seen through the aperture fixed to the headrest so that only the center parts of the rods are seen against the white background, thus avoiding monocular clues. The central rod *F* is fixed in its position; the other rods, seen in peripheral vision, are movable by handles below their channels. The task of the observer is to set the peripherally seen rods so that they all appear in a frontoparallel plane with the fixated rod.

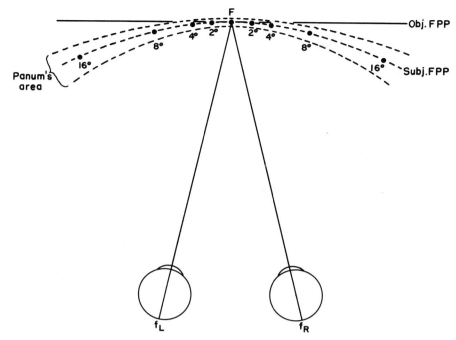

Fig. 7-2. Schematic presentation of the horopter and Panum's area of single binocular vision. The drawing is not to scale. The dots indicate the setting of the horopter wires seen in peripheral vision at the indicated distances required to make them appear in a frontoparallel plane (FPP). All points connecting the dots lie, therefore, on the horopter. The area in back and in front of the horopter, also demarcated by dotted lines, indicates Panum's area of single binocular vision.

ployed. The simplest and most practical, and the only one to be discussed here, is the criterion of frontoparallel appearance of the rods.

The observer is asked to place the movable rods in peripheral vision in such a manner that all rods appear to him in a plane parallel to his forehead or equidistant with the fixated rod. To the *subjective frontoparallel plane,* so determined, corresponds a plane, curved toward the observer, in which the rods are located in physical space. This curved plane is known as the *horopter* (Fig. 7-2). It represents the locus of the object points in physical space that, for the given fixation distance, stimulate corresponding retinocortical elements. All object points located in the horopter appear to lie in a flat plane. The corresponding elements have *zero stereoscopic value.*

When the peripheral rods are in front or behind the horopter plane, they are imaged on disparate retinal elements and are, therefore, seen in diplopia. But this is true only if the displacement of the peripheral rods exceeds a certain distance. At a 45-cm fixation distance the observer can advance or recede the rods a millimeter or two without their doubling up. However, they appear then *in front of or behind* the fixation rod. In other words, there is relative depth difference between the two visual objects, the fixated rod (as frame of reference) and the peripheral rod, which has been moved. They are seen in *stereoscopic depth*. The limits within which it is possible to see singly with disparate elements were defined already over 100 years ago by the Danish physiologist Panum. They have often been measured since. The narrow regions around the horopter plane within which there is a single binocular vision has been termed Panum's area (Fig. 7-2).

This lengthy introduction was required to make clear the physiological mechanism by which stereopsis comes about. *Stereopsis results from the fusion of horizontally disparate retinal stimuli located within Panum's area of single binocular vision.* The qualification of "horizontal" is necessary since vertical disparity is not productive of stereoscopic effects. If there is *temporal* disparity the disparately imaged object appears nearer than the frame of reference; if there is *nasal* disparity it appears *in back* of it. This is analogous to the behavior of the nearer and farther objects in physiological diplopia.

Another way of defining stereopsis is preferred by physicists and engineers. Owing to the horizontal separation of the eyes (the interpupillary distance), each eye, for geometrical reasons, receives a slightly different image of a solid object, say a cube. There is a disparity (in terms of the physiologists) or a *parallactic angle* (in terms of the physicist). This notion of a parallactic angle quantitizes the disparity and is very useful in the construction of instruments of various kinds concerned with stereopsis, but it does not advance our understanding of how sensory fusion of the two unequal retinal images results in a three-dimensional percept.

Certain properties of stereopsis essential for the understanding of its physiological basis and practical determination will now be discussed. Using again the rod apparatus as a model, it is found that the more a peripheral rod is displaced toward or away from the observer, the greater is the depth effect. In other words, *the depth effect is proportional to the disparity.* This may seem self-evident for a three-dimensional model, but it is applicable also to the two-dimensional tests that are in general clinical use for the determination of stereoscopic function.

In defining stereopsis it was stated that stereopsis results from the fusion of disparate retinal images. While this is generally true, fusion is not absolutely required for stereopsis. Even in diplopia a stereoscopic judgment can be made to a degree.[2] This may be established with the horopter (rod) apparatus by placing one movable rod in front of the fixated central rod until it appears in diplopia. A second movable rod is now aligned with the first rod. If the first rod is just barely seen in diplopia—that is, if it is close to the fixated rod—the setting can be made with relatively high accuracy. The farther the first rod is from the fixated rod, the worse is the accuracy of the setting of the second rod, until finally the alignment is made by chance. It is no longer made on the basis of stereopsis. The accuracy of stereoscopic settings is greatest at the horopter, where a minimal displacement is perceived as a depth difference. Therefore, while the horopter itself denotes the region of zero stereopsis, it is at the same time *the region of highest stereoscopic sensitivity.* This point has importance for the physiological theory of stereopsis.

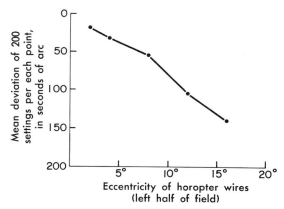

Fig. 7-3. The mean deviation of the setting of the horopter apparatus wires 2, 4, 8, 12, and 16 degrees to the left of the fixated wire is used to indicate the decrease of the stereoscopic threshold in peripheral vision. It is possible to do this since the horopter is the region of highest stereoscopic sensitivity. (From Burian, H. M.: Docum. Ophthal. 23:18, 1967.)

The quantitative relationship between disparity and depth judgment indicates that there is a minimum disparity beyond which there is no stereopsis. In other words, there is a *stereoscopic acuity*.

Highly trained observers have been found in laboratory experiments to respond to limiting angles as low as 5 to 7 seconds, and even 2 seconds, of disparity. Military services requiring stereopsis for acceptance of a candidate place the limit at 15 to 17 seconds. In clinical practice 20 to 40 seconds may be considered as standard stereoscopic acuity.

Stereoscopic acuity is a measure of a person's sensitivity to disparate retinal stimulation within Panum's area of single binocular vision. Clearly, there must be some relation between the minimum separable and stereoscopic acuity. And, indeed, there is. In a subject with normal vision and normal binocular cooperation, the stereoscopic acuity decreases from the center to the periphery of the retina (Fig. 7-3). Artificial reduction of the vision of one eye to 0.1 makes stereopsis impossible. However, except for extreme conditions, there is no absolute dependence of stereopsis on acuity. It has been shown experimentally that reduction of vision in one eye with neutral filters to 0.3 does not materially raise the stereoscopic threshold.[4] Clinical evidence points in the same direction. Patients with unilateral functional amblyopia may respond to disparate stimulations much smaller than one would expect from their visual acuity. And the fact that a patient has a visual acuity of 6/6 in each eye and has fusional amplitudes does not automatically ensure that he has also stereopsis. Such patients suppress selectively disparately imaged stimuli within Panum's area but respond to larger disparities with *motor fusion*.

All this points to a certain independence of stereopsis within the binocular system. It is, therefore, misleading to think of stereopsis as the third or "highest" degree of fusion, while labeling absence of stereopsis in the presence of fusional

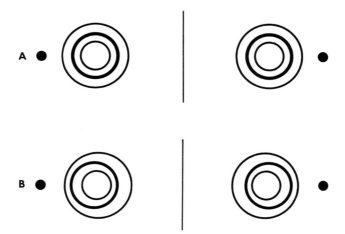

Fig. 7-4. Stereoscope targets. **A,** Concentric circles, fused image flat. **B,** Inner circles displaced, heavy circle temporally (nasal disparity), inner circle nasally (temporal disparity). Fused image seen in depth, small circle in front, black circle in back of outer circle. The black dots in **A** and **B** are fiducial marks.

amplitudes as the "second" degree of fusion. This classification should be dropped.[5]

Since there is a stereoscopic threshold, stereopsis cannot work beyond a certain critical distance. This distance has been variously computed, depending on the threshold selected, as being between 125 and 200 meters or more. Stereopsis is, of course, most effective at lesser distances. This is an important consideration in how a subject handles problems involving depth perception.

There remains an important characteristic of stereopsis to be discussed. The stimulation of horizontally disparate retinocortical elements results not only in fusion with depth perception; there is also a *shift in visual directions,* such that the visual object, seen in depth, is also seen in the visual direction of the corresponding element, relative to which the stimulation is disparate.

Let us consider two pairs of concentric circles. When placed in a haploscope or stereoscope so that each eye sees one set of circles, they appear in binocular view as a single set of flat, concentric circles (Fig. 7-4). If the inner, smaller circles are displaced toward or away from each other, the inner and outer circles appear to be eccentric in monocular view. But when viewed binocularly, the inner circles appear not only singly and in front or in back of the outer circle but also *concentric with it.* This situation is schematically presented for three points in Fig. 7-5. Thus the fused stereoscopic image is seen in the visual direction of the outer circles that are its frame of reference. This startling phenomenon of an *assimilation of visual directions* is of the essence of stereopsis. Without it there is no stereopsis. It also has implications for the clinical use of stereoscopic targets.

One can now go further and investigate what happens when other stimuli are added to the stereogram.[6] If one marks the vertical diameter of the larger

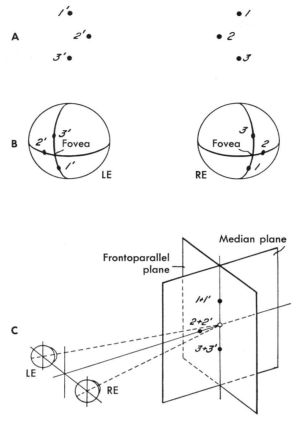

Fig. 7-5. Schematic presentation of shift in visual directions with stereopsis. **A,** Stereoscopic target, represented by three dots. **B,** Dots *1* and *1'* and *3* and *3'* lie on corresponding retinal meridians; dots *2* and *2'* are imaged in temporal disparity. **C,** In the fused image all three dots lie in the median plane. (From Burian, H. M.: Docum. Ophthal. **516:**169, 1951.)

circle (Fig. 7-6, *A*) a continuous line is seen in the fused image, situated in the plane of the large circle. This occurs because the lines are imaged on corresponding meridians of the retinas and they are, therefore, seen in identical visual directions and in the same plane as the large circle that serves as frame of reference. If one now marks in another stereogram the vertical diameters of the small circles (Fig. 7-6, *B*) in the same manner, one again sees in the fused image a continuous vertical line, but this time in the plane of the small circle. The vertical marks fall on disparate retinal meridians, but they are fused and are seen in the visual direction of the corresponding meridians that serve as frame of reference, just as are the small circles themselves.

But if one marks, in a third stereogram, the vertical diameters of both the small and the large circles so that corresponding and disparate retinal meridians are stimulated simultaneously, one observes that the fused image presents one

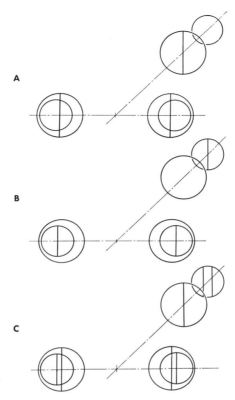

Fig. 7-6. Simultaneous stimulation of corresponding and noncorresponding meridians. **A,** Corresponding vertical meridians stimulated by vertical lines are fused and seen in the plane of large circles. **B,** Noncorresponding vertical meridians stimulated by vertical lines are fused and seen in plane of small circles. **C,** Vertical lines in circles stimulating simultaneously corresponding and noncorresponding meridians cannot be both fused. Either the vertical meridians of the large circles are fused, as shown in the figure, or, with change in convergence, the vertical meridians of the small circles are fused. (From Burian, H. M.: Docum. Ophthal. **516:**169, 1951.)

single vertical line in the plane of the small circle (Fig. 7-6, *C*). If one changes convergence, the diameters of the small circles can be made to be seen singly, but the diameters of the large circles will appear in diplopia. It is never possible to see the diameters of both large and small circles single *at the same time*.

Many modifications of this simple experiment are possible. They all lead to the same conclusion that the fusion of disparate retinal stimulations within Panum's areas and the assimilation of corresponding centers of the areas are stimulated at the same time. It is as if *the direct pathways from the corresponding elements had to be free from impulses* in order to permit excitations reaching them indirectly (from disparate elements) to go through.

These observations lead us to a brief discussion of the *neurophysiological basis of stereopsis.*

The existence of a strict anatomical retinocortical point-to-point relationship has been denied, and with seeming justification. The arborization of the neural connections of the visual system at all levels is such that each retinal receptor or group of receptors is potentially connected with a number of cortical cells. Yet, an orderly physiological relationship is a functional necessity and does indeed exist. This relationship cannot be entirely rigid. Within limits, and to meet requirements of specific stimulus situations, the arrangements must be flexible enough to allow transmission not from one visual receptor (or group of receptors) to one and only one cortical cell (or group of cells). The assimilation of the visual directions in stereopsis is a good physiological example for such a mode of impulse transmission.

A possible explanation for the physiological point-to-point relationship and its flexibility can be found in Lorente de No's old model of the retinocortical relationship.[7] He rejected the avalanche theory of synaptic transmission of Cajal and Herrick and assumed instead that the impulses were funneled from the retina to the cortex. This funneling process would come about as shown in Fig. 7-7.

A retinal element R4 on which the light stimulus is centered would receive maximum stimulation, whereas the elements R2, R3, and R5, R6, to each side of R4, would receive stimuli of decreasing intensity. The impulses from R1 and R7 being subliminal for the cells of the lateral geniculate body, only the impulses from R3, R4, and R5 would proceed to the cortical cells for which the impulses from R2 and R6 would be in turn subliminal. This leaves the retinal element R4 from which the impulses are transmitted or "funneled" to the cortical element C4. Presumably, the corresponding partner of R4 in the other eye would convey impulses in a similar manner to the same cortical cells C4. In this way single vision with corresponding retinocortical elements would come about.

The situation would be different with disparate stimulation of the two retinas. This type of stimulation would induce mechanisms of inhibition and facilitation such that impulses from the disparate elements would be shunted to the "direct line" R4—C4. As a consequence, there would be again a fused image

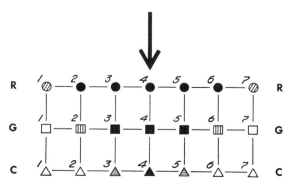

Fig. 7-7. Schematic presentation of retinocortical point-to-point relationship, according to theory of Lorente de No.[7] Numbers *1* to *7* represent adjacent cells in retina *(R)*, lateral geniculate body *(G)*, and primary visual cortex *(C)*. (From Burian, H. M.: Docum. Ophthal. **516**:169, 1951.)

but at the same time the information would be conveyed that the stimuli did not originate in R4. This adds the new quality of stereopsis to vision.

The model presented offers a possible description of why the simultaneous stimulation of the center of reference and of the center of the disparately imaged stimuli is rejected, as in the example with the circles. The "direct line" R4—C4 is busy, as it were, and cannot carry additional information.

Lorente de No's concept was based essentially on morphologic observations. Very recently electrophysiological studies, employing microelectrode techniques, have given evidence for the existence of cells in the cortex that respond selectively to horizontally disparate stimulations of the retinas. Barlow and collaborators[8] and Nikara and collaborators[9] have found such cells in the visual cortex of cats. In the macaque monkey Hubel and Wiesel[10] have discovered cells in area 18 that do not respond to stimulation from either eye but fire maximally when a horizontal disparity of 30-minute arc is introduced. It seems likely that these cells in the cat and the macaque monkey play a role in stereopsis.

In man the techniques used in animals are not applicable. However, with the techniques of visually evoked cortical responses, Regan and Spekrejse[11] and Fiorentini and Maffei[12] have demonstrated that the amplitude of the evoked potential is lower when flat patterns are viewed and higher when the targets are presented stereoscopically.

For the present it is difficult to relate these electrophysiological data to the psychophysically observed stereoscopic behavior in man. But there seems to be little doubt that the very exciting new findings will eventually lead to a full understanding of the neurophysiology of stereopsis.

MONOCULAR (NONSTEREOSCOPIC) CLUES TO SPATIAL ORIENTATION

Stereopsis, the relative localization of objects in depth, can only come about in binocular vision. It is based on a physiological process derived from the organization of the sensory visual system. It is not acquired through experience; it is unequivocal and inescapable.

But stereopsis is restricted to relatively short visual distances and is not the only means we have for spatial orientation. The second set of clues, the monocular or experiential clues, plays an important role in man's estimation of the relative distance of visual objects. These clues are active in monocular as well as binocular vision. They are the result of experience, are equivocal, and are subject to interpretation. It is by means of these clues that a monocular patient improves his depth perception in the course of time, as mentioned earlier in this chapter. Some 50 or 60 years ago there was considerable doubt whether such a relearning could take place, but there is no question that it does in fact occur.

The most important monocular clues are the following.

Motion parallax

When one looks at objects, some of which are closer than the others, and moves one's head or body in a plane parallel to the plane of these objects, one notes an apparent movement of the objects such that the farther objects appear to make a smaller excursion than the nearer objects. This differential angular velocity creates a strong depth impression and is considered to be the most powerful nonstereoscopic clue to depth perception.[13-15] Everyone makes much use of it in daily life. The ophthalmologist, employing direct ophthalmoscopy, moves his head sideways to judge whether there are depressions or elevations in the fundus of an eye. The difference in parallactic movement—for example, of the retinal blood vessels—gives a compelling picture of the different levels in the retina or optic nerve.

Parallactic movements come about when objects sweep with differential angular velocities across the retina not only when the head or body are moved actively but also when they are passively moved. Such a passive movement occurs when one is in a moving vehicle. Tschermak[14] considers this to be of importance in spatial orientation, for example, when riding in a car. But he emphasized also that the differential angular velocities of the retinal images created where one moves one's eyes rather than one's head has no effect on spatial localization, since voluntary eye movements compensate for differences in localization.

Laboratory studies of motion parallax can also be performed by keeping the head steady and moving the objects.[15] It has been shown in such studies, as well as in those in which head movements were employed,[14] that there is a threshold differential angular velocity with which the objects must sweep across the retina to produce a depth effect and that the threshold for vertical movements is approximately twice that for horizontal movements.

Linear perspective

Object points having a constant distance appear to subtend smaller and smaller angles as they recede from the subject, ending to go to a so-called vanishing point (Fig. 7-8, *A*). Railroad tracks that are in fact parallel seem to approach each other in the distance. The foreshortening of horizontal and vertical lines is one of the most powerful monocular clues for depth perception. In urban surroundings such monocular clues abound and are very active. They are absent in other surroundings, such as the underbrush of a forest. Linear perspective is among the most useful tools for the creation of three-dimensional impressions on a two-dimensional surface and has been employed extensively by painters since the Renaissance.

If one keeps oblique lines on purpose parallel in a drawing (Fig. 7-8, *B*) the upper end appears wider than the lower end but also farther away. Placing objects that are supposed to appear more distant on a higher level is a device frequently used by painters prior to the introduction of linear perspective.

Overlay of contours

Configurations whose contours are interposed on the contours of other configurations provide impelling distance clues. An object that interrupts the contours of another object is generally seen as being in front of the object with incomplete contours. This, too, is a clue made use of in realistic paintings to indicate relative distances.

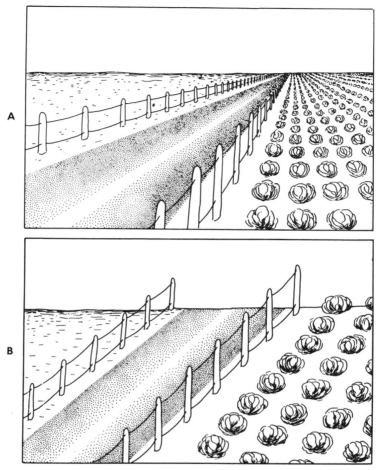

Fig. 7-8. Linear perspective. **A,** Correctly drawn perspective, with parallel lines converging toward a vanishing point and proper size reduction of objects being farther from observer. **B,** Appearance when lines are maintained parallel and all objects are shown equal in size. (From Moses, R. A.: Adler's physiology of the eye: clinical application, ed. 5, St. Louis, 1970, The C. V. Mosby Co.)

Size of known objects

If the size of two objects is known to us, we can judge the relative distance of these objects by their apparent size. If an object that we know to be smaller appears to be larger than the other, we judge it to be nearer.

Distribution of highlights and shadows

Highlights and shadows are potent monocular clues. Since the sunlight comes from above, we have learned that the position of shadows is helpful in determining elevations and depressions—the relative depth—in objects. This is very

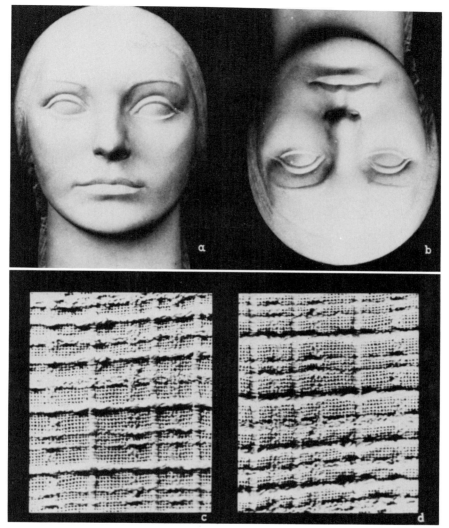

Fig. 7-9. Effect of highlights and shadows. *a,* Sculptured head, photographed with light coming from above. *b,* Same photograph as in *a,* inverted. Some flattening is noted, but nose is not seen as trough. *c,* Piece of cloth, photographed with light coming from above. Horizontal ridges, with shadows below, stand out sharply. *d,* Same photograph as in *c,* inverted. Ridges appear as troughs, with shadows placed above. (From Burian, H. M.: J. Assoc. Med. Illustrators 9:4, 1956.)

impressively shown in Fig. 7-9, in which a photograph of a piece of cloth is photographed by throwing light on it in such a way that horizontal threads in the tissue appear as ridges (Fig. 7-9, *c*). In another copy of the identical photograph turned 180 degrees, the ridges appear as troughs (Fig. 7-9, *d*).

The inversion can occur because nothing in our experience prevents it from happening. But in the photograph of a sculptured portrait head the inversion of the print does not have the same effect (Fig. 7-9, *a* and *b*). Some observers may note a general flattening in the inverted print, but a nose can never be seen as a trough.

Aerial perspective

"Aerial perspective" is the term used for the influence of the atmosphere on contrast conditions and colors of more distant objects. The bluish haze of more distant mountains is an example.

INTERACTION OF STEREOSCOPIC AND MONOCULAR CLUES

The impression of three dimensionality imparted by the nonstereoscopic clues is a judgment, an interpretation. This implies that false judgments are possible, and such is indeed the case. It also implies that this impression depends on past experience, as does every judgment. It is in the nature of the nonstereoscopic clues that they are experiential and that they can be meaningful only when they are capable of being related to past experience of the organism.

All this does not mean that nonstereoscopic monocular clues are less important in everyday life than are stereoscopic clues. Normally the two work hand in hand, one enhancing the effect of the other. But this is not always the case. If one introduces into stereograms confusing clues—that is, monocular clues that conflict with stereoscopic clues—fascinating observations can be made.

Not everyone reacts in the same fashion to such stereograms. Some people are more responsive to disparate stimulation (stereoscopic clues), whereas others respond more readily to monocular clues. These differences result both from physiological peculiarities, or actual abnormalities, of the visual system and from past experience. It is clear that an observer who for years has done laboratory experiments in stereopsis will be particularly responsive to stereoscopic clues.

Many years ago I devised an experimental setup by which it was possible to estimate the extent to which a person gave weight in his judgments to stereoscopic and nonstereoscopic clues.[16]

When a person with normal binocular cooperation is provided with a lens that magnifies the image of one eye in the horizontal meridian (a so-called size lens at axis 90 degrees), a disparity is introduced. If this disparity is within limits, a stereoscopic effect is produced in the sense that objects on the side of the eye wearing the lens are seen farther back, those on the other side closer (Fig. 7-10). Using the horopter (rod) apparatus discussed before, placing of a size lens in front of one eye results in a tipping of the subjective frontoparallel plane around the fixation point, the half of the field on the side of the eye wearing the lens being farther back, the other half farther forward than when no lens is worn.

In order to correct for this, or in order to see the rods again in a frontoparallel plane, the observer must displace the rods in the opposite direction. The horopter is now tipped so that it is closer on the side of the eye with the magnified image, farther back in the other half of the field. In persons with normal binocular vision this tipping is linear with respect to the amount of magnification within the permissible limits of disparity and is therefore a mea-

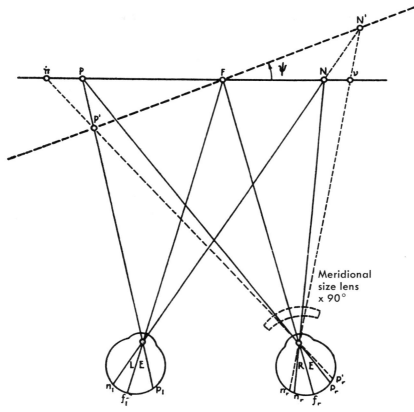

Fig. 7-10. Effect of meridional size lenses at axis 90 degrees on a frontoparallel plane. The size lens causes the section *PN* of the frontoparallel plane to be magnified to π to ν on the right retina. Fusion $P\pi$ causes *P* to appear in front and $N\nu$ in back of the frontoparallel plane. The whole plane has rotated around the fixation point *F*. For the plane to appear again fronto-parallel *P* has to be placed back and *N* placed forward a corresponding amount. (From Burian, H. M.: Arch. Ophthal. [Chicago] **30:**645, 1943.)

sure of the introduced stereoscopic effect. In doing such experiments, as in all horopter determinations, nonstereoscopic clues are carefully avoided. One can now, on purpose, introduce nonstereoscopic, perspective clues to assess their effect on the settings.

For this purpose I used a board, rotatable around its central vertical axis, provided with an appropriate design (Fig. 7-11). The observer had first to set this board so that it appeared to him in his subjective frontoparallel plane. Meridional size lenses at axis 90 degrees with magnification properties of 0.5% to 3% or 4% were then placed in front of one eye, say to the right. With each lens the observer had to set the board anew so that it would appear to be in his subjective frontoparallel plane. In this fashion nonstereoscopic clues (the target) and stereoscopic clues (the disparity induced by the lens) were offered. If a

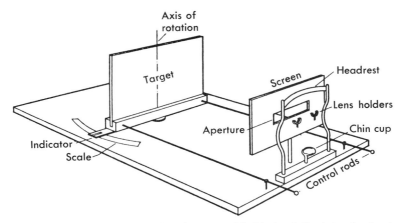

Fig. 7-11. Rotating plane apparatus. The observer, with his head fixed in the headrest, looks at the target, which carries perspective patterns and is rotatable by control rods around a vertical axis. Lens holders are provided to insert meridional size lenses. The observer's task is to maintain a frontoparallel position of the rotary target plane. (From Burian, H. M.: Arch. Ophthal. [Chicago] **30:**645, 1943.)

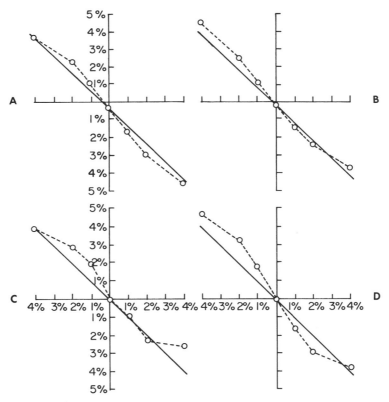

Fig. 7-12. Settings of the rotating plane apparatus of four different observers (**A** to **D**) with a series of meridional size lenses at axis 90 degrees. These observers follow the introduced disparity clues rather well. Abscissa, magnification introduced by lenses. Ordinate, angle of rotation required to see the rotating plane in frontoparallel position with lenses of increasing magnification. Right half, lens in front of OD; left half, lens in front of OS. (From Burian, H. M.: Arch. Ophthal. [Chicago] **30:**645, 1943.)

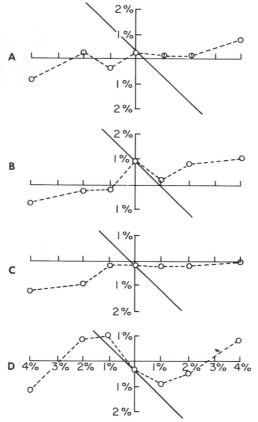

Fig. 7-13. Settings of rotating plane apparatus of four different observers (**A** to **D**) with a series of meridional size lenses at axis 90 degrees. These observers do not follow the introduced disparity clues but rely for their judgment on the perspective clues, although they follow the disparity clues normally in the absence of monocular clues. Presentation is same as in Fig. 7-11. (From Burian, H. M.: Arch. Ophthal. [Chicago] **30:**645, 1943.)

person gave great weight to stereoscopic clues, the settings of the board would more or less approximate the setting of the rod apparatus, free of monocular clues (Fig. 7-12). Persons who relied more or less on perspective clues would follow the lens-induced disparity only to a degree or not at all (Fig. 7-13). In the latter subjects no added lens would produce a setting of the board different from the one made without the lens, although the same person would make the correct settings with the rod apparatus. This device then provided valuable information about the response that an individual would make when offered a choice between stereoscopic and nonstereoscopic clues.

CLINICAL AND OTHER PRACTICAL ASPECTS
OF DEPTH PERCEPTION

The only function of depth perception that is at present being investigated routinely in clinical practice is the function of stereopsis. There are no tests for the quality of orientation in the third dimension by means of nonstereoscopic clues. This situation has not always prevailed. Some 60 and 70 years ago such testing aroused considerable interest and discussion, especially with regard to the questions of whether and to what extent monocular individuals could regain better visuomanual coordination following, for example, an accident in which one eye was lost. This was considered significant with a view to estimating the possible loss of working capacity of such individuals.

It is regrettable that tests involving nonstereoscopic clues do not exist at this time. For while it is unquestionable that the possession of stereopsis represents the optimal visual situation toward which the visual system has evolved, nevertheless stereopsis is not indispensable for the functioning of man in his three-dimensional environment. The nonstereoscopic clues supply man's needs significantly in this respect. For far distances they are alone operative. They are no less active in near vision, but here the stereoscopic clues allow for a more refined, quantitative localization of visual objects in the third dimension. This is, of course, important, and it has been often emphasized that in the highly industrialized culture of our day stereopsis is increasingly important. This may be questioned. Much close work, from threading a needle to the assembling of electronic parts, is largely a matter of sighting, although stereopsis may be of considerable help, and certain tasks cannot be performed by persons lacking stereopsis. Every x-ray man who does not have stereopsis, and his ophthalmologist, are only too well aware of this. But, aside from such highly specialized tasks, nonstereoscopic clues have great usefulness. It will be suggested later in this chapter how motion parallax may be employed to ascertain the quality of a person's depth perception.

TESTING FOR STEREOPSIS

There are, generally speaking, two reasons why an ophthalmologist tests for stereopsis. In patients with neuromuscular anomalies of the eyes he often wants to know whether or not the patient responds to disparate stimulations and, if so, what his stereoscopic threshold is. Second, the ophthalmologist has on occasion to certify that a person has a certain level of stereopsis required for specific activities or occupations.

Testing for stereopsis may be performed with equipment ranging from very simple devices to complex laboratory apparatus. There are two groups of tests that the ophthalmologist may employ, tests making use of two-dimensional objects as test material (targets placed in a major amblyoscope or stereoscope, vectograph cards) and three-dimensional devices (three-rod machines, Verhoeff stereoptor, Hering falling bead test). The former group is in most widespread use.

Using two-dimensional test objects

Tests making use of two-dimensional test objects (targets, cards) must incorporate two essential features. The two eyes must be dissociated—that is, each eye must be presented with a separate field of view—and each of the two fields or targets must contain elements imaged on corresponding retinal areas, to serve as frame of reference, and disparately imaged elements to be fused and seen stereoscopically. In addition, they should contain fiducial marks to check whether both eyes are used simultaneously.

The targets may be opaque or transparent and may be used in a major amblyoscope or stereoscope. Both devices have in common that the fields of view are mechanically separated, that they are set optically at infinity, and that they employ exchangeable targets. The major amblyoscope has the advantage that its arms can be set at the angle of deviation of the patient, thus allowing control of the retinal area being stimulated. It can be achieved similarly with the stereoscope by the use of prisms, but this procedure may not be as accurate and the distortions induced by prisms may become bothersome.

The number and variety of targets are limited only by the ingenuity of the designer and user, but standard sets of targets and cards are commercially available for the different major amblyoscopes and stereoscopes. Targets of interest in the present context are especially those containing objects with differing amounts of disparity (for example, the Keystone DB_6 card) so that they appear to be at different relative depth distances. The object having the least disparity that is seen in depth by the patient denotes his stereoscopic threshold.

A useful clinical application can be made of the simple stereogram consisting of eccentric circles, one set seen with each eye (Fig. 7-4). If the patient reports that he sees two fiducial marks and two circles, but not in depth, one should inquire whether the two circles are concentric. They cannot be seen concentrically unless they are seen also stereoscopically. If they are seen eccentrically, one may now ask whether the inner circles is closer on the right or closer on the left of the outer circle. The patient's answer determines whether the disparate elements are suppressed in the right eye or the left.

In vectograph cards the eyes are dissociated optically. A vectograph consists of Polaroid material on which the targets are so imprinted that each target is polarized at 90 degrees with respect to the other. When the patient is provided with properly oriented Polaroid spectacles, he sees each target separately with the two eyes. At the present time only one such test is commercially available, the Titmus Stereotest. In this test a gross stereoscopic pattern, representing a housefly, is provided to orient the patient and to establish whether he has gross stereopsis (threshold: 1,000 seconds). In testing young children it is necessary to ask questions that the child will understand. One may, for example, ask the child to get a hold of the wings of the fly. If the child sees them stereoscopically, he will reach above the plate. It is amusing to watch the child's startled look when he does so. It is indeed an eerie feeling not to have a tactile sensation of a seen object. Some children, though they have stereopsis, will touch the wings on the plate because they "know" that they are there. One must explain to them that one does not inquire about what the child knows, but what he sees.

The Polaroid test also contains three rows of animals, one in each row being imaged disparately (thresholds: 100, 200, and 300 seconds, respectively). The child is asked which one of the animals stands out. The animal figures contain a misleading clue. In each row one of the animals, correspondingly imaged in two eyes, is printed heavily black. A child without stereopsis will name this animal as the one that stands out.

Last, the Polaroid test provides nine sets of four circles arranged in the form of a lozenge. In this sequence the upper, lower, left, or right circles are disparately imaged at random with thresholds ranging from 800 to 40 seconds. If the child has passed the other tests, it is now asked to "push down" the circle that stands out, beginning with the first set. When the child makes mistakes or finds no circle to push down, the limits of his stereopsis are presumably reached.

In administering this test—and for that matter, any test for stereopsis that requires that separately presented images be fused—it is essential not to rush the patient. It takes at times quite a while before the stereoscopic effect is noted. Also, it is on occasion wise to go back to patterns with grosser stereopsis that the patient has passed. He will often have a more definite impression of three dimensionality than he had the first time.

If one has doubts whether the patient does in fact see stereoscopically or not, one may occlude one eye and inquire whether there is a difference in appearance, say of the housefly, with one or both eyes open. And since only horizontal disparity produces stereopsis, one can also turn the plate 90 degrees, which should block out the stereoscopic effect.

Some people believe that the vectograph circle test is unreliable, because one can note that the displaced circles are "different" when looked at without the Polaroid spectacles. This is evident with the circles displaced by 800 to 200 seconds. Some keen observers with very high acuity can go almost all the way. The assumption that this makes the test unreliable is erroneous. When the eyes are provided with Polaroid spectacles, both disparate images are either perceived —in which case they are fused and seen stereoscopically—or one of them is suppressed and there is no stereoscopic effect. This is entirely different from the observations made without the Polaroid spectacles.

Because of the simplicity of administration, the Titmus Stereotest is at present most widely used by ophthalmologists who bother at all with the testing of stereopsis. However, one is not always justified in stating simply that "the patient has no stereopsis," that is, that he has no sensitivity for disparate stimuli, on the basis of this test alone. It must be kept in mind that the vectograph test is a test for near vision. Some patients suppress disparate stimulations at near but respond to them in distance fixation or vice versa. This is usually the case when the deviation is intermittent at one fixation distance and heterotropic at the other. It is always wise to supplement the vectograph test with a stereoscope or major amblyoscope test adapted for distance fixation.

How should the stereopsis determined with any of these tests be recorded? Cards and vectographs that attempt to quantify stereopsis are graded in different ways. Some use artificial scales (such as the Sheppard scale); many speak of percentage of stereopsis, assuming a certain threshold to mean 100%. All this is misleading and arbitrary. The only proper way to record stereopsis is by the amount of disparity incorporated into the target. It is unequivocal and it should be generally understood, when it is stated that a patient had stereopsis with a threshold of 400 seconds or 100 seconds or 40 seconds, or whatever the threshold may be.

It remains to be discussed what use the ophthalmologist may make from the information obtained in testing for stereopsis.

Although stereopsis is not "the highest degree of fusion" but a qualitatively different visual sensation, refined stereoscopic sensitivity can exist only if the patient accepts simultaneous stimulation of the two foveal regions. Some ophthalmologists use stereoscopic tests to determine whether or not patients with very small or intermittent deviations have foveal suppression. If the stereoscopic threshold is low enough, they conclude that there is no foveal suppression. A positive result is certainly conclusive but a negative result does not necessarily mean that the foveal impressions are completely suppressed. There are patients who accept all but disparate retinal stimuli.

In my hands a positive stereoscopic response of a patient with a neuromuscular anomaly of the eyes, at any fixation distance and in any part of the binocular field, is of paramount importance prognostically and in directing the treatment. The finding makes it mandatory that every effort be made, surgically and nonsurgically, to restore to the patient full binocular cooperation with stereopsis at all fixation distances and in every part of the field.

If all tests show that a patient has no potential for sensory cooperation, it is useless to strive for anything more than a good cosmetic result. The patient cannot achieve more and is well served if his appearance is normalized. But if there is actual binocular cooperation, be it ever so restricted, one is in duty bound to attempt a functional improvement unless one pays only lip service to our proclaimed goal of functional cures.

Employing three-dimensional test objects

Only one three-dimensional test is readily available commercially. This is the Verhoeff stereoptor. This test consists of a small, handy box containing some free-standing black wires placed at different distances and seen against a background of diffusing glass, illuminated from behind. Some of the wires are wider

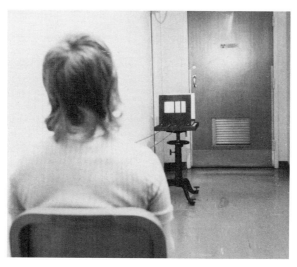

Fig. 7-14. Subject making observation on Howard-Dolman depth perception device. (From Howard, H. J.: Amer. J. Ophthal. 2:656, 1919.)

than others, introducing a misleading clue. There are four different wire positions, which are seen through apertures on the front of the device. The instrument may be inverted, thus giving a total of eight different wire positions. The observer should be able to see the wires in proper depth at 1 meter. If the stereoscopic threshold of the patient is lower, the instrument will have to be approached correspondingly, thus increasing the visual angle and therewith the disparity. It is recommended that one record the stereoacuity obtained with this instrument in a manner analogous to the Snellen notation. Then if the patient recognizes the position of the wires correctly at 1 meter, his stereoscopic acuity is represented by D/100 or 20/20, if at 50 cm it is noted as 20/40, and so on.

A test devised in 1919 by Howard,[17] generally known as the Howard-Dolman test, is essentially an application of the two- and three-rod tests first used by visual physiologists of the nineteenth century. It consists of two black rods placed 6 meters from the observer or patient. The rods are seen through an aperture so arranged that the observer sees only the central part of the rods against a white background. One rod is fixed. The second rod may be moved remotely by the subject who attempts to position his rod exactly opposite the fixed rod. A millimeter scale allows measurement of how precisely this alignment was accomplished. Positioning to within an arbitrary distance in 75% of twenty trials is considered success. The observer's head may be secured by a comfortable headrest, thus avoiding motion parallax (Fig. 7-14).

Finally, a test should be mentioned, introduced 100 years ago by Hering, in

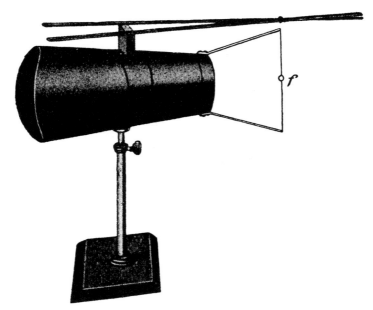

Fig. 7-15. Hering's apparatus for the falling bead test. The observer looks into the black tube at left, fixating the bead f. The experimenter drops beads of varying sizes at different distances from f on a cloth.

which an instantaneous depth judgment is required of the patient. The test is the so-called falling bead test. The patient looks into a short black tube (Fig. 7-15) that carries at its farther end a wire with a fixation mark. Beads of varying sizes are dropped on a cloth at different distances from the fixation mark and the minimum distance is determined at which the patient states correctly whether the bead fell in front or in back of the fixation mark.

To determine the quality of monocular depth perception

As has been stated before, there are no clinical tests specifically designed to test the ability of a one-eyed person to localize objects in the third dimension. Since it would be valuable if such tests were available, some suggestions how this could be done will be made in this section.

Motion parallax is the most powerful clue to depth perception and at the same time the most convenient clue to investigate depth perception of one-eyed individuals. Tschermak[14] conceived for this purpose a device that he termed a "parallactoscope." It consisted of a frame carrying a central fixed set of vertical wires with a set of vertical wires to each side, movable in an anteroposterior direction. The position of the movable wires could be judged with great accuracy in binocular observation by a person endowed with stereopsis. The accuracy was reduced to chance in a monocular individual whose head was fixed. But his

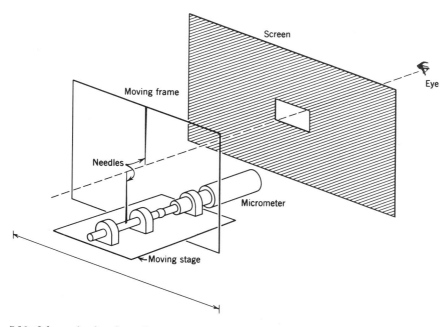

Fig. 7-16. Schematic drawing of apparatus used by Graham and others[15] for the testing of motion parallax. The needle driven by the micrometer is adjustable in a plane parallel to the line of sight. The subject adjusts this needle until it is in the same plane as the fixed, upper needle. The moving stage, containing the needles and accessory equipment, moves in the frontal plane. (From Graham, C. N.: Visual space perception. In Graham, C. N., editor: Vision and visual perception, New York, 1965, John Wiley & Sons, Inc., p. 504.)

accuracy in localizing the position of the wires improved greatly when he was permitted to move his head sideways.

Instead of introducing head movements, Graham and collaborators[15] proposed a device in which the head was kept steady but the target was moved. The field of view contained two needles seen as opaque against the field illumination, one stationary, and the other movable at a constant speed in a plane perpendicular to the line of sight of the subject (Fig. 7-16). The movable needle could be displaced away from or toward the observer, thus producing monocular movement parallax when the two needles were at unequal distances from the observer's eye. The task of the observer was to set the two needles in such a way that both needles appeared to be in the same plane or so that no movement was perceptible.

Graham and his collaborators devised their apparatus to be able to investigate various parameters, such as differences in size of the moving objects, the effect of luminance, rate of movement of the objects, and axis of movement of the objects, on monocular movement parallax. This device could be standardized and produced in a compact form for the purpose of clinical testing of motion parallax and its effect in monocular individuals.

While such a device is at present not available, the ophthalmologist can use to this end any of the three-dimensional tests for stereopsis described earlier by allowing or encouraging head movements while the test is being performed.

If he wishes, the ophthalmologist can construct, or have constructed, a very simple device designed by Cords[13] as far back as 1913 for the specific purpose of testing the effect of motion parallax on spatial localization. I had this done and found the apparatus quite useful.

The device (Fig. 7-17) consists of a box 30 cm long and 20 cm wide and high.

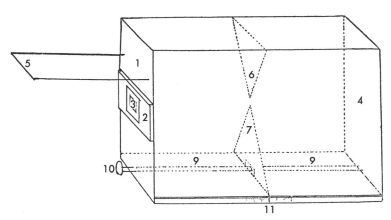

Fig. 7-17. Apparatus to test effect of motion parallax devised by Cords.[12] *1*, Front wall of box; *2*, carrier for various apertures *(3)*; *4*, diffusing glass wall; *5*, rod to indicate placement of forehead; *6*, fixed black triangle; *7*, black triangle movable on rod *9*; *10*, knob for rod *9*; *11*, index and scale indicating position of lower triangle.

The back end of the box is formed by diffusing glass, the front end carries an arrangement permitting the insertion of various apertures. In the middle of the box is suspended a fixed black triangle to which corresponds a second, movable triangle. This lower triangle can be placed at varying distances from the fixed triangle, the distance being indicated by a marker and scale on the outside of the box. A metal bar fixed to the outside of the box places the patient's forehead at desired distance without fixating it. The test consists in placing the lower triangle at varying distances from the upper fixed triangle and to find within what range the observer or patient reports that position correctly in a predetermined number of trials.

It is self-evident that this test can be used also to determine the stereoscopic threshold in binocular individuals. Monocular patients are encouraged to use horizontal head movements to aid them in spatial orientation. Cords even recorded these head movements on a kymographic drum with a pen attached to a band placed on the patient's head.

In applying his test Cords[13] found that persons with normal binocular vision whose one eye he occluded made larger errors than people who had been monocular for 1 year or more. The best and speediest responses were obtained in monocular individuals who had been one-eyed since early youth.

REFERENCES

1. Readers interested in further reading on this subject are referred to the following works: Tschermak-Seysenegg, A.: Introduction to physiological optics (translated by P. Boeder), Springfield, Ill., 1952, Charles C Thomas, Publisher; Ogle, K. N.: Researches in binocular vision, Philadelphia, 1950, W. B. Saunders Co.; Ogle, K. N.: Optical space sense. In Davson, H., editor: The eye, New York, 1962, vol. 3, Academic Press, Inc.; Graham, C. H.: Visual space perception. In Graham, C. H., editor: Vision and visual perception, New York, 1965, John Wiley & Sons, Inc., p. 504.
2. Burian, H. M.: Studien über zweiängiges Tiefensehen bei örtlicher Abblendung, Graefe, Arch. Ophthal. **136:**172, 1936.
3. Burian, H. M.: Discussion of paper by Schubert, G.: Physiologie des Binocularsehens, Docum. Ophthal. **23:**18, 1967.
4. Matsubayashi, A.: Forschungen über die Tiefenwahrnehmung IX, Acta Soc. Jap. **42:**1920, 1938; German abstract, Ber. Ges. Physiol. **112:**291, 1939.
5. Burian, H. M.: The place of peripheral fusion in orthoptics, Amer. J. Ophthal. **30:**1005, 1947.
6. Burian, H. M.: Stereopsis, Docum. Ophthal. **5/6:**169, 1951.
7. Lorente de No, R.: Studies on the structure of the cerebral cortex, II. Continuation of the study of the ammonic system, J. Psychol. Neurol. **46:**113, 1934.
8. Barlow, N. C., Blakemore, C., and Pettigrew, J. D.: The neural mechanism of binocular depth discrimination, J. Physiol. **193:**327, 1967.
9. Nikara, T., Bishop, P. O., and Pettigrew, J. D.: Analysis of retinal correspondence by studying receptive fields of binocular single units in cat striate cortex, Exp. Brain. Res. **6:**353, 1968.
10. Hubel, D. H., and Wiesel, T. N.: Stereoscopic vision in macaque monkey: cells sensitive to binocular depth in area 18 of the macaque monkey, Nature **225:**41, 1970.
11. Regan, D., and Spekreijse, H.: Electrophysiological correlate of binocular depth perception in man, Nature **252:**92, 1970.
12. Fiorentini, A., and Maffei, L.: Electrophysiological evidence for binocular disparity detectors in human visual system, Science **169:**208, 1970.
13. Cords, R.: Bemerkungen zur Untersuchung des Tiefenschätzungsvermögens, III. Die Verwertung der parallaktischen Verschiebung durch Einäugige, Z. Augenheilk. **32:**34, 1914.

14. Tschermak-Seysenegg, A.: Über Parallaktoskopie, Arch. Ges. Physiol. **241:**455, 1938/1939.
15. Graham, C. H., and others: Factors influencing thresholds for monocular movement parallax, J. Exp. Psychol. **38:**205, 1948.
16. Burian, H. M.: Influence of prolonged wearing of meridional size lenses on spatial localization, Arch. Ophthal. (Chicago) **30:**645, 1943.
17. Howard, H. J.: A test for the judgment of distance, Amer. J. Ophthal. **2** (Series 3):656, 1919.

CHAPTER 8 *Electrophysiological measurements**

ALBERT M. POTTS

Unlike much of the preceding material, the information contained in this chapter is not intended to be a "how-to-do-it" section. Rather its purpose is to give enough basic information to the practitioner so that he may judge the desirability of using electrophysiological methods to further his clinical diagnosis. It is desired, moreover, to present the basic principles on which these electrophysiological measurements rest, so that further developments in this rapidly changing field may be understood and utilized where appropriate.

ELECTRORETINOGRAM
Basics

The electroretinogram (ERG) is a series of small voltage changes measured across the globe when a light stimulus is presented to the eye. It was first described by Holmgren in 1865.[1] All vertebrates and many higher invertebrates exhibit the ERG, and it was demonstrated quite early that the measured change was entirely caused by the retina itself. The isolated frog retina was used in this demonstration by Kühne and Steiner[2,3] and in recent years the isolated human retina has also been made to produce an ERG.[4]

Electrode

In the intact human subject an electrode system has been arrived at that allows examination of the ERG with minimum patient discomfort. This system utilizes a contact lens electrode making electrical contact with the cornea (and allowing passage of the light stimulus because of its transparency). It also involves an "indifferent" electrode, frequently on the forehead. The net effect of this electrode arrangement is measurement of the voltage across the globe. The forehead electrode is electrically the same as if it were behind the globe, the orbital tissues being the "connection" between the forehead electrode and the eye (Fig. 8-1).

The type of contact lens has changed from the molded scleral lens originally

*Supported in part by U.S. Public Health Service Research Grant No. EY-00212 from the National Eye Institute, Bethesda, Md., and by the L. L. Sinton Trust Research Grant.

187

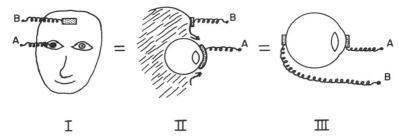

Fig. 8-1. Connection of ERG electrodes. The potential moves across a contact lens electrode *A* and an "indifferent" forehead electrode *B*. *I* is equivalent to *II*, which shows how the forehead is electrically connected to the back of the globe. This can be depicted diagrammatically as in *III*.

introduced by Riggs[5] to the low-vacuum contact lens of Henkes,[6] or the Burian-Allen lens[7] with integral speculum. With proper topical anesthesia and the use of high-viscosity methylcellulose as contact vehicle, an examination of 30 to 60 minutes with no patient discomfort is standard. Beyond this time corneal erosions with attendant discomfort become relatively common.

Recording

The voltage change picked up by the electrode system described previously reaches only 250 to 1,100 μv for normal subjects and less in disease, so for any serious study an amplifying device is required before being able to record the ERG. In clinical electroretinography the almost universal custom has been to use a condenser-coupled amplifier with a moderately long time constant. Indeed, the commercial availability of such amplifiers designed for EEG recording is one of the factors that has made the procedure clinically feasible. Recording has been attempted with pen writing devices, but mechanical inertia is a distinct detriment to the reproduction of fast, low-amplitude changes. Much more satisfactory is photography of the trace on a cathode-ray oscilloscope. Polaroid photography makes this recording process very easy but somewhat more expensive than conventional photography. With such equipment all of the ERG features to be described are measurable except for the very slow c-wave.

Light stimulus

Study of the off-effect (see Fig. 8-4) requires a stimulus lasting several hundred milliseconds. The great convenience of the electronic flash tube whose stimulus duration is about 1 msec has led clinical electroretinographers to adopt it and to sacrifice study of the off-effect. The additional advantage of the electronic flash is that with proper circuitry it can be fired repetitively and can be used as a flicker source of value in the study of photopic responses.

Some attention has been devoted to how the stimulus is delivered to the eye. For clinical purposes it is desirable that the stimulus cover a wide enough area so that extremely accurate fixation is not required of the subject. Generally clinicians have been satisfied with a flash tube in a reflector at a distance of

1 to 2 feet from the eye. It has been shown by Echte and Papst[8] that there is a measurable increase in response if the entire field of vision of the subject is stimulated ("ganzfeld" stimulus). Additional equipment is required to achieve this—either an inside illuminated stimulus sphere[9] or a contact lens with a pre-placed 100D lens.[8] So far most clinical electroretinographers have been reluctant to make these innovations, but the changes are simple enough to warrant their adoption. It should be added that for additional constancy of results the pupil should be dilated, possibly with addition of an artificial pupil. The only exception to this is in using the Echte and Papst contact lens in which the 100D lens passes the light as a tiny bundle through the normal pupillary aperture.

Adaptation

Amplitude of all ERG waves increases with dark adaptation, so for maximum amplitude some 30 minutes of adaptation is necessary. Since the total tolerance to most contact lens electrodes is 30 to 60 minutes, waiting for complete adaptation in a routine clinical examination is impractical. Various compromises have been used. A common expedient is to measure the scotopic ERG after 10 minutes of dark adaptation, by which time 75% or better of the final effect has been reached. A second expedient is to adapt to a very low light level rather than complete darkness.[10] Under the conditions I have used in the past—a field at a brightness of 7×10^{-2} ft-L—complete adaptation is achieved in 7.5 minutes and the b-wave amplitude is 90% of that obtained at 30 minutes adaptation in the dark.

The amplitude of the ERG of a subject adapted to room light levels and above is quite small. Hence in the past it has not been customary to study the morphology of the photopic ERG. However, additional information has been obtained by studying the flicker ERG. Amplitude of flicker response, although small, can be measured in normal persons. The resultant ERG is said to be composed of a negative a-wave and a positive off-effect.[11] The flicker ERG is detectable at frequencies above the subjective flicker fusion frequency. There is good evidence, such as that obtained with a rod achromat by Gouras and Gunkel,[12] that above circa 8 Hz the flicker ERG is mediated by retinal cones rather than rods. Thus the flicker ERG at higher frequencies is a valid measure of function of the photopic retina.

Summation

With high-intensity stimuli the scotopic ERG is remarkably reproducible. Nevertheless, small details are better seen and amplitudes are more precisely measured if some type of summation of a number of records is used. If one is interested in determining the ERG threshold to low-intensity stimuli, this is even more true. The present availability of special purpose computers for signal averaging puts averaging capabilities in the hands of a number of electroretinographers. To take an example at random, a paper by Auerbach[13] shows several types of signal averaging. The use of the general purpose digital computer for analysis of serial ERG's, including signal averaging, is in its infancy[10] but is destined to play an important role in the future.

MORPHOLOGY
Dark-adapted ERG

Demonstration of all the ERG subcomponents ever described requires a direct current (DC) amplifier, a very high-intensity and constant light source, and a shutter that delivers a square wave pulse of several seconds' duration. None of this equipment is practical for clinical use. As was mentioned before, the usual clinical ERG recording is done with an alternating curent (AC) amplifier and a flash tube stimulus that makes it impossible to record c-wave and off-effect. The possible remaining features are each capable of examination (Fig. 8-2) and

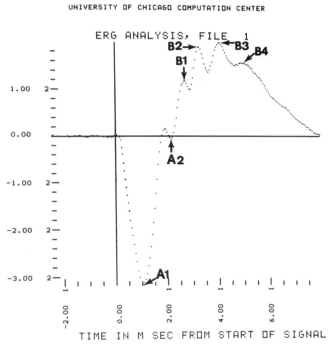

Fig. 8-2. The high-intensity scotopic electroretinogram. With high-intensity flash stimuli and dark adaptation the ERG shows at least six maxima and minima. The figure shows a computer averaged sum of five stimuli given 2 minutes apart. *A1,* Shortest latency, first negative deflection, sometimes called *photopic a-wave* or *late receptor potential. A2,* Second negative deflection, sometimes called *scotopic a-wave.* At lower intensities this deflection is at the same level as A1. It is the increase in negativity of A1 which is responsible for their separation here (see Fig. 8-3). *B1,* First positive deflection. (The positive wave at A2 and the negative components at B1 to B4 have not been studied.) This appears only as a slope change at intensities 1 log unit lower and not at all with still weaker stimuli. *B2,* Second positive deflection. This has been called *photopic b-wave* and *x-wave.* At lower stimulus intensities it appears where A2 is seen here. *B3,* Third positive deflection. This is the deflection that was the sole positive response at low intensities (see Fig. 8-3). It is the *scotopic b-wave. B4,* Fourth positive deflection, seen at high stimulus intensities only. It is a slope change at 1 log unit less intensity. B1 through B4 are labeled oscillatory potential (see text).

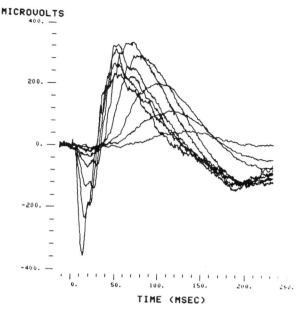

MICROVOLTS

Fig. 8-3. Composite of scotopic ERG's (AH 20CT71 #16). Nine levels of stimulus are shown varying over an intensity range of 10,000 times. Each trace is the sum of ten responses at a given intensity. Note the decrease in b-wave latency for the five lowest intensities; the increase in b-wave amplitude for the five lowest intensities; the increase in a-wave amplitude for the four highest intensities; and the lack of change in height above the baseline for the four highest intensities.

some attention has been given to them, as will be described later. However, it should be appreciated that early in the study of the clinical ERG many of the present refinements of technique were not available or not appreciated and in many studies nothing was measured except b-wave amplitude. The large amount of information about the b-wave in disease is therefore as much a function of its ease of measurement as of its importance. The two a-waves, the "x-wave" or b_1 seen at high intensities, and the multiple remaining b-waves, part of which constitute the "oscillatory potential," can all be measured reproducibly with adequate technique, and each has been assigned clinical significance. The effect of increasing stimulus intensity on the scotopic ERG is shown in Fig. 8-3. In addition, flicker response to increasing frequency of stimulus can be measured and gives additional information on the cone system.

ORIGIN OF THE COMPONENTS OF THE ERG
b-Wave

At the very lowest light levels that give a response with the clinical equipment described, the ERG consists of a single, positive deflection of relatively long latency. As stimulus strength is gradually increased it is apparent that this deflection is the cornea-positive scotopic b-wave. If one measures the ERG in an experimental animal and simultaneously records the optic nerve discharge, it is clear that the optic nerve is conducting an impulse milliseconds before the b-wave reaches its peak.[14] Thus the b-wave is not in the main line of the visual impulse but must be considered an after-potential. Its magnitude reflects stimulus magnitude but represents a relatively late correlate of vision. Physiological evidence from experimental animals locates the b-wave origin in a retinal region external to the ganglion cells and internal to the receptor cells.[15,16] It is perhaps not surprising, then, that recent work by Miller and Dowling locates the major b-response in the Müller cells of the retina.[17] The research in question used the *Necturus* (a salamander) as an experimental animal, but there is no reason to disbelieve extrapolation of this finding to the human case. It fits the known facts to have the b-wave generated by a glial cell not directly involved in transmission of the visual impulse but whose late restorative changes could easily reflect the magnitude of that impulse.

a-Wave

When the b-wave is abolished by giving glutamate[15] or by occluding the retinal circulation without disturbing the choroidal circulation,[16] what remains on the record is a negative response that returns only to the baseline. This is the pure a-wave and it undoubtedly arises from the receptor cells.

At the very lowest stimulus intensities the a-wave does not exist. The a-wave appears at intensities 2.0 to 2.5 log units above b-wave threshold and is soon seen to have two components. The component with the lower latency is cone-dependent and that with the longer latency appears to be rod-dependent. They are frequently known as a_1 and a_2, respectively.

With the onset of the a-wave one sees the negative-going a-wave and positive-going b-wave opposing one another, so b-wave amplitudes become meaningless at this point for clinical purposes. The a-wave amplitudes continue to be linear with log intensity, but the b-wave is best studied at these stimulus intensities by means of its latency rather than its amplitude. The a-wave latency changes very little and does not appear to be a promising field for clinical study.[10]

Because of this static b-wave and growing a-wave at high intensities, some writers have redefined the b-wave so that it is measured by them from the lowest negative point to the highest positive point on the tracing. Although this helps to salvage a low-amplitude ink-writer record, it introduces additional confusion into an already confused nomenclature. On balance it seems far more desirable to measure a-deflections negative to the baseline and b-deflections positive to the baseline, always remembering that after the onset of the a-wave, b-wave amplitudes at still higher intensities are of no practical value.

"Early receptor potential"

By speeding up the recording rate and by using very intense stimuli and light-shielded microelectrodes in experimental animals, a very early potential change was described in laboratory animals by Cone[18] and by Brown and Murakami.[19] There is a tiny positive deflection followed by a larger negative deflection. The latency of these changes is very small, indeed, compared to the remainder of the ERG, so that relatively fast sweep speeds and relatively high amplification are required. Brown and Murakami named this phenomenon the "early receptor potential" or ERP. For the sake of consistency, if not logic, Brown renamed the a-wave the "late receptor potential." One must be on guard against confusion from this source.

Experiments have shown that the early receptor potential can be obtained from the isolated retina and has an activity curve that parallels that of rhodopsin.[18] However, the eye cup with retina removed gives a similar electrical response to a light flash, and here the cell of origin appears to be the pigment epithelium cell[20] and the photopigment appears to be melanin.[21] With the best of techniques and under laboratory conditions it is still impossible to completely eliminate an artifact in the record caused by the photoelectric effect on a metal electrode at high stimulus levels. There is considerable question as to whether any of the early receptor potentials reported under *clinical conditions* are true bioelectric potentials. It seems to me that the burden of proof lies upon the clinical electroretinographer to demonstrate that he is measuring an eye potential, not an artifact, and to demonstrate clinical values for the measurement.

"Oscillatory potential"

With high-intensity stimuli one sees one or more wavelets following the two standard b-waves. These have been named the "oscillatory potential" by Yonemura and co-workers.[22] The implication of this term is that the wavelets are caused by a single generator and are superimposed upon a b-wave of major proportions. That this is erroneous is demonstrated in the latency studies of Potts and associates.[10] In fact, the "b-wave" is an assembly of components with individual amplitudes and latencies. Each of the components must be studied separately and the oscillatory notion should be abandoned. However, there are significant clinical implications of the wavelets. These will be discussed later.

Analysis

The earliest thorough analysis of the components of the ERG, and the basis for a recent Nobel Prize award, was that of Granit.[23] It was shown by Granit that in the dark-adapted retina of higher vertebrates electrical excitatory processes prevail over inhibitory ones. He labeled this type the "E retina" (excitatory) as opposed to the "I retina" (inhibitory) of lower vertebrates. In each type he applied varied pharmacological agents and was able to show that the ERG was

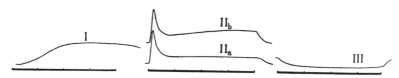

Fig. 8-4. The Granit analysis of the ERG into its component parts. Process I, the c-wave; abolished by light adaptation. Process II, the b-wave; abolished early in ether anesthesia. Two alternatives are shown. Process III, the a-wave and off-effect (d-wave); remaining after light ether anesthesia, abolished by further ether administration. (From Granit, R.: J. Physiol. **77:**220, 1933.)

a composite of three separate processes. Process I (PI) accounts for the slow late cornea-positive rise in potential that we have called the c-wave. Process II (PII) is the fast cornea-positive rise that accounts for the b-wave. Process III (PIII) is the rapid cornea-negative response causing the a-wave and whose late relaxation is responsible for the off-effect. This analysis is shown in Fig. 8-4. It does not account for "early receptor potential" or "oscillatory potentials" but it is still valid for the major ERG components.

CLINICAL SIGNIFICANCE OF THE ERG

There are several ways to look at ERG changes in eye disease. The theoretician wishes to know all diseases in which ERG changes occur because such information may tell him new things about the ERG. The practicing clinician is interested only in those disease changes that are best demonstrated by electroretinography and where simpler psychophysical office procedures fail. These are the only cases where referral for an ERG examination makes sense. In the following we will try to make it clear which diseases are in the second category.

b-Wave

As we mentioned previously, by far the greatest amount of clinical electroretinography has concerned b-wave amplitude recorded under variably controlled conditions. Even though the b-wave may well originate in the Müller cells, it accurately reflects stimulus intensity over much of its amplitude range. The b-wave amplitude also is a measure of the number of intact "functional units" in operation as the result of the stimulus. For the purposes of this discussion let us consider the "functional unit" as whatever combination of receptors is required to activate a bipolar cell, which in turn will activate a ganglion cell and cause an optic nerve impulse. The more units are active, the more surrounding Müller cells will respond with the after-potential that we call the b-wave and the greater the b-wave amplitude. That this is true has been demonstrated experimentally in the human by Brindley and Westheimer.[24]

It follows that any disease interrupting the activity of large numbers of functional units will cause decrease of b-wave amplitude. It makes no difference whether the interruption occurs near the site of generation of these potentials in the bipolar cell layer (as in occlusion of the central retinal artery) or whether the damage is to photoreception (as in retinal detachment)—the result is the same. The amplitude of the b-wave is decreased and the amount of decrease is related to the amount of retina destroyed. A destructive chorioretinitis will similarly reduce b-wave amplitude if the destruction is extensive enough.

In all of these diseases, diagnosis may be reached swiftly without resort to the ERG. However, where damage is extensive but diffuse it is less easily detected by other means. In the extreme instance of heredoretinal degenerations the b-wave change is often the first detectable sign of disease. It is worth considering the special applications in more detail.

Heredoretinal degenerations

For a detailed treatment of this complex subject one should consult a treatise such as that of Franceschetti, François, and Babel[25] or, less satisfactorily,

Duke-Elder and Dobree.[26] Electrophysiological interest in this area begins with the observation of Karpe[27] that patients with retinitis pigmentosa have no ERG response. This refers to the typical autosomal recessive form. It became clear later that the dominant form of the disease shows a measurable but diminished response. Only rare exceptions among the cases of recessive retinitis pigmentosa show a measurable ERG.[28] In any case the magnitude of the change is a certain guide to the examiner, allowing differentiation between pigmentary retinopathy and other diseases such as inflammations that cause pigmentary changes that might be confused with true retinitis pigmentosa.

Flecked retina syndrome

A second large category of disease in which the ERG plays a useful diagnostic role is the collection of related disease that Krill and Klien have brought together under the inclusive heading of "flecked retina syndrome."[29] The components of the syndrome have been described by previous authors as "fundus flavimaculatus," "fundus albipunctatus," and "drusen." Ophthalmoscopy shows fundus changes that may strongly suggest the presence of this syndrome. Confirmation is given by delayed dark adaptation accompanied by delay in the time required for the scotopic b-wave to reach its normal amplitude.

Congenital amaurosis of Leber

The ophthalmologist is frequently asked for an opinion about the vision of an infant suspected of having poor acuity. When ophthalmoscopy shows a "pepper-and-salt" fundus and a pale disk, the differential diagnosis rests between congenital amaurosis of Leber and rubella syndrome with high probability. The distinction is easily made with electroretinography. The former disease nearly always shows no ERG (92% of cases reviewed by Alström and Olson[30]). Rubella, despite widespread pigmentary changes, ordinarily leaves a normal ERG.[31] One should note the variants of congenital amaurosis where fundus changes other than the typical "pepper-and-salt" appearance are present. They are all characterized by b-wave loss.[31]

Toxic retinopathies

Historically a number of substances administered as drugs have caused pigmentary retinopathy with b-wave changes.[32] At present only two of these are still being administered to patients—they are thioridazine and chloroquine (and its close relatives). The first drug appears to be safe if an upper dosage level is not exceeded. The second appears to be toxic only if given in total cumulative dose of greater than about 100 gm and over a period of more than a year. Even with these conditions fulfilled, it is not possible to predict which chloroquine patients will show toxic effects. However, with either drug, when toxicity occurs, an extensive pigmentary retinopathy may supervene and in the early stages profound attenuation of the b-wave is the rule. The curious observation that thioridazine toxicity causes equally profound loss of dark adaptation and chloroquine toxicity does not is useful in diagnosis.[33]

Congenital hemeralopias

The subject of congenital hemeralopias is reviewed by Franceschetti and associates.[34] Essential hemeralopia with dominant inheritance is characterized by the presence of b_1 and the absence of b_2. The recessive form of the disease shows an a-wave and a small photopic b. The other tests of visual function are likely to be more valuable in the diagnosis of this disease than electroretinography, but the ERG may have confirmatory value. In Oguchi's disease the physical findings are distinctive. Electroretinographically there is typically a small but present b_1 and no b_2.

a-Wave

One should recall that when stimulus intensity is great enough to elicit both a- and b-waves, these potentials oppose one another. Thus, in entities characterized by pathological reduction of the b-wave, the unopposed a-wave can appear larger than normal. Clinical electroretinographers describe this as a "negative" electroretinogram and sometimes as a "supernormal" a-wave. The most clear-cut instance already cited occurs in occlusion of the central retinal artery. Siderosis bulbi is another disease entity in which one can find this phenomenon. In neither instance is the ERG likely to be an indispensible diagnostic aid. In the case of Oguchi's disease, a large a-wave is typical because of the lack of b-wave opposition.[34]

"Oscillatory potential"

There has been relatively little study of oscillatory potential because it has been identified only recently. As stated previously, there is good evidence that the postulated periodicity has to do only with accidental spacing of multiple ERG components. Whatever the origin of the wavelets, they can be measured, and it is the opinion of two research groups that the "oscillatory potential" is markedly and selectively reduced in diabetes even in the eyes of subjects who show no retinopathy ophthalmoscopically and in the presence of an otherwise normal ERG.[35,36]

Flicker

We mentioned previously that flicker above about 10 cps is referable to the retinal cones. Since cones are present throughout the retina except in the extreme periphery, this measurement should not be interpreted as an investigation of foveal function. At least one clinical condition represents absence of cones throughout the retina. This is the case of the rod monochromat whose inheritance pattern is autosomal recessive. The typical amblyopia plus achromatopsia in these patients is adequately diagnostic, but in addition and for what it is worth flicker response is not detectable above 10 cps (Hz).[37] Further, the photopic single flash response is absent or measurably diminished.

It is evident from the foregoing that although the ERG represents the mass activity of a large number of cells, and although in many retinal diseases ophthalmoscopy is enough for diagnosis, there are a number of diseases where the ERG is useful or even indispensible. Inherited pigmentary retinopathies, toxic retinopathies, flecked retina syndrome, and congenital amaurosis of Leber are some of these.

VISUAL EVOKED RESPONSE (VER)

It was demonstrated nearly 40 years ago that a flash of light caused an electrical response at the visual cortex of an experimental animal.[38] However, conversion of this finding obtained with intracortical electrodes into a clinical examination on an intact human subject had to await the advent of a signal averaging system that would let the 5-μv response be detectable amid 10 μv of random electrical and biological "noise." For reasons detailed later, routine employment of the VER in the clinic is still in the future. However, vigorous research is being done in a number of clinics. The promise of clinical usefulness is so great that it cannot be ignored. Even now research establishments are producing early clinical results.

The equipment required for recording the VER is standard electroencephalographic equipment plus a special purpose digital computer and a standard light stimulus that may be repeated at least once a second. For an excellent discussion of equipment and methods for VER see the book of Perry and Childers.[39] To obtain a readable record it is necessary to summate a number of responses, sometimes several hundred. To make the summation meaningful only time-corresponding points of each response must be added. That is, all response points 5 msec after the stimulus should be summed to give a single point on the final record, all response points 10 msec from the stimulus should be similarly

SINGLE RESPONSES   SUMMED RESPONSES

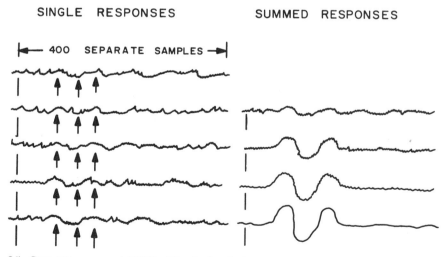

Fig. 8-5. Computer-averaged EEG's. The basis of signal averaging as used in VER recording. The separate samples on the left have information that is no larger than the "noise" level but that occurs at the same relative time (arrows) in relation to the stimulus. When these records are summed by the computer, the signal grows and the noise averages out as shown on the right.

summed, all 15-msec points, and so on. The result will be a record where real signal components will add to one another to make an easily discernible deflection—positive or negative—and the "noise," being random, will cancei out and result in negligible deflection (Fig. 8-5). A diagram of our VER system is shown in Fig. 8-6.

Electrodes

Ordinary ERG electrodes are adequate. Nonpolarizable electrodes are not required, but the commercially prepared silver–silver chloride self-adhesive electrodes are convenient. Maximum response appears to be obtained between occiput and the parietal area. Lateral placement causes surprisingly little augmentation or diminution of response with monocular stimulation. Positioning in the midline, for example at O_z to P_z (according to international nomenclature), is an adequate arrangement for either eye.

The light stimulus that has proved most practical so far is the electronic flash. There are some theoretical reasons why a sine-wave light stimulus should make for easier analysis,[40] but until now clinical convenience has favored the short flash. The subject of stimulus is inseparably bound up with the problem of what is responding to produce the VER. The available evidence suggests that the VER represents the sum of potential changes undergone by at least the first neuron in the visual cortical chain and possibly some unknown number of subsequent ones. It is evident that the VER must reflect pathological conditions in the entire visual system from retina to cortex. It is conversely apparent that the VER will reflect the overall organization of the visual system from retina to cortex. Thus in direct contrast to ERG, where amplitude is a function of number of cells stimulated, the VER takes cognizance of the importance of central vision

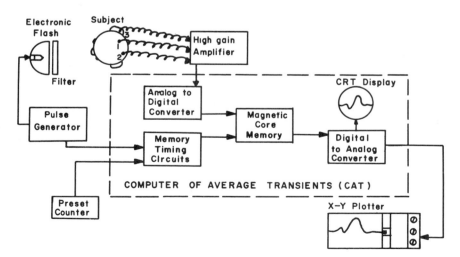

Fig. 8-6. Block diagram of apparatus for recording VER. A number of special purpose computers are now available for this job. Properly configured general purpose computers are also satisfactory.

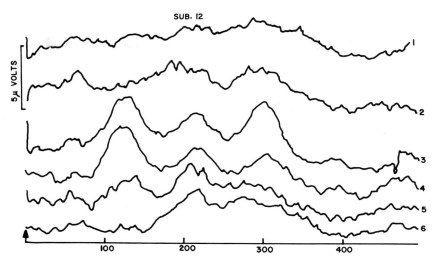

Fig. 8-7. Effect of centration of stimulus on VER (0.06-degree red stimulus, 690 mμ). *1,* Stimulus 1.75 degrees temporal to fixation; *2,* stimulus 1.15 degrees temporal to fixation; *3,* central fixation; *4,* stimulus 0.6 degree nasal to fixation; *5,* stimulus 1.15 degrees nasal to fixation; *6,* stimulus 1.75 degrees nasal to fixation. (From Potts, A. M., and Nagaya, T.: Invest. Ophthal. 4:303, 1965.)

to the overall system. VER amplitude is greater in the photopic retina. A tiny central target is enough to cause a relatively large response whereas decentering of the same target abolishes response.[41] The acuity findings which the VER reflects are shown in Fig. 8-7.

In addition to the conventional flash stimulus, we should consider a somewhat different type of stimulus—the checkerboard stimulus. There are a number of ways in which the 5 central degrees of the visual field may be stimulated with a checkerboard pattern. One can build the stimulator so that the checkerboard alternates at each cycle—white squares becoming black and vice versa. With a little care in balancing, one can ensure that this alternation results in no net change in illumination.[40] Thus one is dealing with an entirely different type of stimulus from the light flash. It works not by momentarily switching on the most central foveal cones with a light stimulus but by causing a change in edge contrast. Under optimal conditions this type of stimulus can elicit a response comparable in amplitude to that caused by a flashing light.

That this stimulus is a function of resolution of the squares can be demonstrated easily. If accommodation is abolished with a cycloplegic, an optimum correction can be found that gives maximum response to a checkerboard of given square size. Less than 1.00D change on either side of the optimum abolishes the response completely.[42] The use of this type of stimulus obviates the necessity for a stimulating ophthalmoscope to place a spot stimulus precisely in the fovea for a noncooperative subject. All that is needed is an alternating checkerboard that fills the visual field. This promises to represent a great simplification for the VER technique.

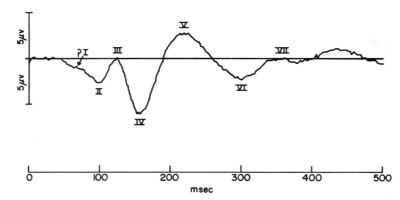

Fig. 8-8. Visual evoked response as obtained at University of Chicago. (Labeled according to Cigánek.)

Typical response

There is still considerable debate over what constitutes a typical VER response. The description with the greatest assurance is that of Cigánek.[43] This author describes six deflections—three positive and three negative—with peak latencies of 40 to 135 msec and amplitudes of 0.9 to 7.1 mv. Fig. 8-8 shows one of our VER results labeled after Cigánek.

The problem is that, although taken overall the VER does have the general characteristics described by Cigánek, the response of a given individual may differ widely from the prescribed norm. It appears that the VER of a given individual tends to remain constant over a long period, but there may be great individual differences from the Cigánek average.[44,45] This suggests that, for clinical use, when one normal pathway is present it can act as adequate control for the side suspected of disease. Where there is a question as to whether both sides are involved, it is considerably more difficult to distinguish an abnormal response from a normal variant. The most constant finding is the presence of Cigánek's waves II, III, and IV. It is by no means clear at present whether the best measure is amplitude from trough of III to peak of IV, or area under a given amount of curve, or some other measure. This is the aspect of clinical VER under study in a number of laboratories, including ours at the present time.

The clinical usefulness of the VER must be understood to be appreciated. The usual clinical psychophysical measurement of visual acuity and visual field are excellent examinations. With the help of an intelligent cooperative adult patient they cannot be surpassed by an electrophysiological method. However, there are numerous instances where visual acuity in particular must be obtained in an infant, a malingerer, or a psychotic adult. This is the task best accomplished by an objective electrophysiological measurement. This is the goal of researchers in the clinical VER. As understanding of the tool increases, improvements will be added. Even now, with a checkerboard stimulus that fills the visual field, we are approaching that goal and can give a good estimate of the vision of an uncooperative subject.

ELECTRICAL EVOKED RESPONSE OF THE
VISUAL SYSTEM (EER)

As mentioned previously, the VER requires the totality of the visual system for its functioning. It would be desirable if similiar objective methods could be devised for stimulation of intermediate structures along the path. Until now central nervous system anatomy has defeated this with one exception—the EER.

For more than 200 years we have known that an electrical pulse to the eye would produce a sensation of light.[46] It seemed reasonable that this sensation could be recorded from the occipital cortex and, indeed, we were able to accomplish this at the University of Chicago.[47] By paying particular care to stimulus intensity and to isolation of the stimulating electrode, it was possible to record the EER from human subjects. By using rats with inherited degeneration of receptor cells, it was possible to demonstrate that the bipolar cells were the site of action of the EER. Thus the visual system was measured beginning one step distal to the receptors.[48] When the EER was determined on patients with retinitis pigmentosa and was compared to the VER on the same patients, it served as a measure of relative damage of bipolar as compared to receptor cells.[49] It is this type of application for which the EER is suited. To date we have not yet succeeded in stimulating the ganglion cell neuron or the geniculocalcarine neuron.

ELECTRO-OCULOGRAM (EOG)

The first discovered bioelectric potential of the eye was the "standing" (DC) voltage across the globe found by Du Bois-Reymond.[50] The major component of this DC voltage originates in the retina and microelectrode investigations in experimental animals have localized the retinal component at the pigment epithelium—receptor cell boundary. Numerous attempts to use the DC potential as a measure of retinal function have failed because of the lack of constancy of absolute measurements. However, the *change* of this potential from light adaptation to dark adaptation as described by Arden and co-workers[51] is reproducible, particularly when eye movement is used to generate the potential difference. Fig. 8-9 shows how the eye forms a dipole with its apex relatively positive to the base. Electrodes are placed near the outer and inner canthus. The subject is required to move his eyes 30 degrees right, then 30 degrees left every 10 seconds for four to five times each minute of the testing period. When the right eye moves temporally, the outer canthus is positive relative to the inner canthus. When the right eye moves nasally, the inner canthus electrode is positive relative to the outer canthus. The type of record generated is shown in Fig. 8-9. The step potentials are averaged both under dark-adapted and light-adapted conditions. The final ratio is expressed as light peak to dark trough. At the University of Chicago the lower limit of normal for this ratio is 2.

Clinical applications

Wherever there is damage to pigment epithelium one may expect to find a decrease in the EOG ratio, and in general this is true. In retinitis pigmentosa,[52] in chloroquine and thioridazine retinopathy,[33] and in choroideremia[53] where pigment epithelium is involved, the EOG is depressed. However, there is some

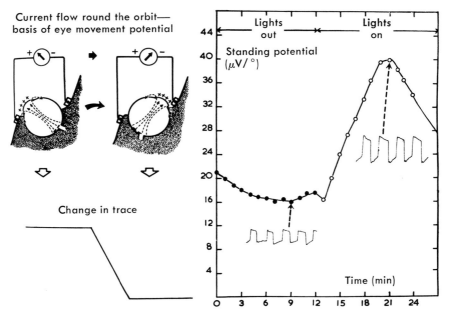

Fig. 8-9. The electro-oculogram. Left portion of this figure shows how with an electrode at each canthus polarity can be reversed as globe is rotated first temporally, then nasally. Right portion of figure shows reproduction of actual trace and its amplitude change from dark to light. (From Arden, G. B., and Fojas, M. R.: Arch. Ophthal. [Chicago] **68:**369, 1962.)

lack of consistency in the degree of depression. For example, it has long been known that the b-wave of the ERG is abolished early in the common (recessive) form of retinitis pigmentosa. Although there are marked abnormalities of EOG in this disease, there are cases where some dark-light change persists.[54] This is despite the fact that the primary disease is presumably in the pigment epithelium, where the EOG is generated, and not in the middle layers of the retina, where the b-wave is generated. In these instances the value of the EOG is chiefly as a confirmatory test rather than a diagnostic one. However, in identifying chloroquine retinopathy by the discrepancy between impaired ERG and EOG and relatively normal dark adaptation,[33] the role of the EOG is more central.

The EOG is reduced in retinal detachment, which is not surprising, and in central retinal artery occlusion, which is surprising.[55] One would not expect an effect at the level of the pigment epithelium from closure of a vessel that supplies only inner retinal layers. This plus the nonparallelism with ERG in retinitis pigmentosa suggests that EOG requires more study. In both detachment and arterial occlusion, visual fields and ophthalmoscopy are likely to be adequate clinical diagnostic measures, and the EOG as presently known will not make a great original contribution.

The EOG is useful in the study of night blindness. It is subnormal in the dominant but not in the recessive form of hereditary night blindness.[56] This makes its use highly important in this area.

In one other category the EOG has some importance; it has been observed by Arden[57] and substantiated at the University of Chicago that certain macular degenerations that seem to be confined strictly to the posterior pole show abnormal EOG's. This is a prime example of how electrophysiological testing can go beyond physical examination in some instances. In those macular degenerations where the EOG is abnormally low, we are evidently dealing with widespread retinal disease of which the only visible portion is macular but whose true extent is shown by the EOG.

To summarize, the EOG is a relatively simple test whose clinical applications have been real but modest until now. In inherited night blindness and in disease of the posterior pole it has unique information to offer. In pigmentary retinopathies—inherited and drug induced—there is useful information to be had. In other diseases that involve widespread retinal destruction, such as vascular occlusions, retinal detachment, and extensive chorioretinitis, it has little to offer beyond what can be had with ophthalmoscopy and psychophysical testing.

SUMMARY

It is evident from the foregoing that the number of electrophysiological procedures for investigation of the visual system is becoming formidable. With the

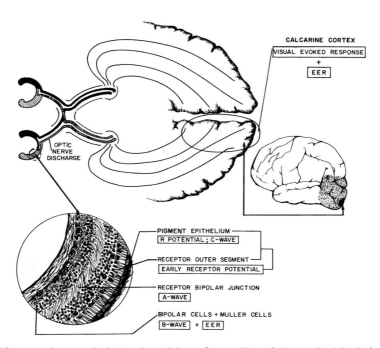

Fig. 8-10. Diagram of anatomical sites for origin and recording of electrophysiological potentials.

help of these procedures, many aspects of the function of the visual system that have been amenable only to psychophysical test methods now can be measured objectively. In the case of some disease entities unique information not otherwise obtainable is given by the electrical approach. A diagram summarizing the anatomical facts about electrophysiological methods is seen in Fig. 8-10.

REFERENCES

1. Holmgren, F.: Method att objectivera effecten av ljusentrych på retina, Uppsala Läkaref, Förh. **1**:177, 1865.
2. Kühne, W., and Steiner, J.: Über das electromotorische Verhalten der Netzhaut, Untersuch. Physiol. Inst. Univ. Heidelberg **3**:327, 1880.
3. Kühne, W., and Steiner, J.: Über electrische Vorgänge im Sehorgan, Untersuch. Physiol. Inst. Univ. Heidelberg **4**:64, 1881.
4. Haschke, W., and Sickel, W.: Das Elektroretinogramm des Menschen bei Ausfall der Ganglienzellen und partieller Schädigung der Bipolaren, Acta Ophthal. **70**(Supp.):164, 1962.
5. Riggs, L. A.: Continuous and reproducible records of the electrical activity of the human retina, Proc. Soc. Exp. Biol. Med. **48**:204, 1941.
6. Sundmark, E.: ERG recording with different types of contact glass, Acta Ophthal. **70**(Supp.): 62, 1962.
7. Burian, H., and Allen, L.: A speculum contact lens electrode for electroretinography, E.E.G. Clin. Neurophysiol. **6**:509, 1954.
8. Echte, K., and Papst, W.: Vorteile der Linsen-Haftschale für die Registrierung des Elektroretinogramms, Acta Ophthal. **70**(Supp.):176, 1962.
9. Berson, E. L., Gouras, P., and Gunkel, R. D.: Rod responses in retinitis pigmentosa dominantly inherited, Arch. Ophthal. (Chicago) **80**:58, 1968.
10. Potts, A. M., and others: The morphology of the human ERG, Eighth Symposium of ISCERG, Pisa, Italy, 1970. In press.
11. Heck, J.: The flicker electroretinogram of the human eye, Acta Physiol. Scand. **39**:158, 1957.
12. Gouras, P., and Gunkel, R. D.: The frequency response of normal rod achromat and myctalope ERGs to sinusoidal monochromatic light stimulation, Docum. Ophthal. **18**:137, 1964.
13. Auerbach, E.: The value of the different components for clinical electroretinography. In François, J., editor: The clinical value of electroretinography, Basel, 1968, S. Karger AG, p. 162.
14. Praglin, J., Spurney, R., and Potts, A. M.: An experimental study of electroretinography: I. The electroretinogram in experimental animals under the influence of methanol and its oxidation products, Amer. J. Ophthal. **39**:52, 1955.
15. Potts, A. M., Modrell, R. W., and Kingsbury, C.: Permanent fractionation of the electroretinogram by sodium glutamate, Amer. J. Ophthal. **50**:901, 1960.
16. Brown, K. T., and Watanabe, K.: Rod receptor potential from the retina of the night monkey, Nature (London) **196**:547, 1962.
17. Miller, R. F., and Dowling, J. E.: Intracellular responses of the Müller (glial) cells of the mudpuppy retina: their relation to b-wave of the electroretinogram, J. Neurophysiol. **33**: 323, 1970.
18. Cone, R. A.: Early receptor potential of the vertebrate retina, Nature (London) **204**:736, 1964.
19. Brown, K. T., and Murakami, M.: A new receptor potential of the monkey retina with no detectable latency, Nature (London) **201**:626, 1964.
20. Brown, K. T., and Crawford, J. M.: Intracellular recording of rapid light-evoked responses from pigment epithelium cells of the frog eye, Vision Res. **7**:149, 1967.
21. Brown, K. T., and Crawford, J. M.: Melanin and the rapid light-evoked responses from the pigment epithelium cells of the frog eye, Vision Res. **7**:165, 1967.
22. Yonemura, D., Tsuzuki, K., and Aoki, T.: Clinical importance of the oscillatory potential in the human ERG, Acta Ophthal. **70**(Supp.):115, 1962.

23. Granit, R.: The components of the retinal action potential in mammals and their relation to the discharge in the optic nerve, J. Physiol. 77(3):207, 1933.

24. Brindley, G. S., and Westheimer, G.: The spatial properties of the human electroretinogram, J. Physiol. **179**:518, 1965.

25. Franceschetti, A., François, J., and Babel, J.: Les heredo-dégénérescences chorio-rétiniennes, Paris, 1963, Masson et Cie, p. 212.

26. Duke-Elder, Sir S., and Dobree, J. H.: System of ophthalmology: X. Diseases of the retina, St. Louis, 1967, The C. V. Mosby Co., p. 577.

27. Karpe, G.: The basis of clinical electroretinography, Acta Ophthal. 24(Supp.):5, 1945.

28. Rubrino, A., and Ponte, F.: The role of electroretinography in the diagnosis and prognosis of retinitis pigmentosa, Acta Ophthal. **70**(Supp.):232, 1962.

29. Krill, A. E., and Klien, B. A.: Flecked retina syndrome, Arch. Ophthal. (Chicago) **74**:496, 1965.

30. Alström, C. H., and Olson, O.: Heredo-retinopathia congenitalis Monohybrida recessiva autosomalis, Hereditas **43**:1, 1957.

31. Francois, J., and De Rouck, A.: Electroretinography in the diagnosis of congenital blindness. In François, E., editor: The clinical value of electroretinography, Basel, 1968, S. Karger AG, p. 451.

32. Potts, A. M.: Clinical usefulness of electrophysiological measurements. In Straatsma, B. R., and others, editors: Retina: morphology, function and clinical characteristics, Berkeley, 1969, University of California Press, p. 545.

33. Krill, A. E., Potts, A. M., and Johanson, C. E.: Advanced chloroquine retinopathy: investigation of discrepancy between dark-adaptation and the electroretinographic findings in advanced stages, Amer. J. Ophthal. **71**((2):530, 1971.

34. Franceschetti, A., François, J., and Babel, J.: Les heredo-dégénérescences chorio-rétiniennes, Paris, 1963, Masson et Cie, p. 1207.

35. Yonemura, D., Aoki, T., and Tsuzuki, K.: Electroretinogram in diabetic retinopathy, Arch. Ophthal. (Chicago) **68**:19, 1962.

36. Simonsen, S. E.: ERG in diabetics. In François, J., editor: The clinical value of electroretinography, Basel, 1968, S. Karger AG, p. 403.

37. Krill, A. E.: The electroretinogram in congenital color vision defects. In François, J., editor: The clinical value of electroretinography, Basel, 1968, S. Karger AG, p. 205.

38. Gerard, R. W., Marshall, W. H., and Saul, L. J.: Cerebral action potentials, Proc. Soc. Exp. Biol. Med. **30**:1123, 1933.

39. Perry, N. W., and Childers, D. G.: The human visual evoked response, Springfield, Ill., 1969, Charles C Thomas, Publisher.

40. Spekreijse, H.: Analysis of E.E.G. responses in man evoked by sine-wave modulated light, The Hague, 1966, Dr. W. Junk N.V.—Publishers.

41. Potts, A. M., and Nagaya, T.: Studies on the visual evoked response: I. The use of the 0.06° red target for evaluation of foveal function, Invest. Ophthal. 4:303, 1965.

42. Potts, A. M., and Hirata, A.: Unpublished data.

43. Cigánek, L.: Die elektroencephalographische Lichtreitzantwort der menschlichen Hirnrinde, Breslau, Bratislava, 1961, Slovakian Academy of Sciences Press.

44. Dustman, R. E., and Beck, E. C.: Long term stability of visually evoked potentials in man, Science **142**:1480, 1963.

45. Werre, P. F., and Smith, C. J.: Variability of responses evoked by flashes in man, E.E.G. Clin. Neurophysiol. 17:644, 1964.

46. LeRoy, C.: Ou l'on rend compte de quelques tentatives que l'on a faites pour guérir plusieurs maladies par l'électricité, Mém. Acad. Roy. Sci. Paris, 1755, p. 60.

47. Potts, A. M., Inoue, J., and Buffum, D.: The electrically evoked response of the visual system (EER), Invest. Ophthal. 7:269, 1968.

48. Potts, A. M., and Inoue, J.: The electrically evoked response of the visual system (EER): III. Further contribution to the origin of the EER, Invest. Ophthal. 9:814, 1970.

49. Potts, A. M., and Inoue, J.: The electrically evoked response of the visual system (EER): II. The effect of adaptation and retinitis pigmentosa, Invest. Ophthal. 8:605, 1969.

50. Du Bois-Reymond, E.: Untersuchungen über thierische Elektrizität, Berlin, 1849, Dielrich Reimer, Andrews & Steiner.

51. Arden, G. B., Barrada, A., and Kelsey, J. H.: New clinical test of retinal function based upon the standing potential of the eye, Brit. J. Ophthal. **46:**449, 1962.

52. Arden, G. B., and Fojas, M. R.: Electrophysiological abnormalities in pigmentary degenerations of the retina, Arch. Ophthal. (Chicago) **68:**369, 1962.

53. Gouras, P.: Clinical electro-oculography. In Straatsma, B. R., and others, editors: Retina: morphology, function and clinical characteristics, Berkeley, 1969, University of California Press.

54. François, J.: The differential diagnosis of tapetoretinal degenerations, Arch. Ophthal. (Chicago) **59:**88, 1958.

55. Nagaya, T.: The standing potential of the eye in vascular and degenerative disease of the retina, Bull. Yamaguchi Med. School **11:**187, 1964.

56. Carr, R. E., and others: Rhodopsin and the electrical activity of the retina in night blindness, Invest. Ophthal. **5:**497, 1966.

57. Arden, G. B.: The relationship between electroretinogram and electro-oculogram. In Schmöger, E., editor: Electrophysiology and pathology of the visual system, Leipzig, 1968, Georg Thieme Verlag, p. 15.

CHAPTER 9 *Assessment of special visual function*

ARTHUR H. KEENEY

"Special functions" in vision are areas in which basic physiology is subject to varied influences that are difficult to standardize. These functions have been subjected to complex or cumbersome laboratory studies, but reliable and efficient clinical techniques have not yet attained familiarity in the testing arena of clinical practice. Assessment of these functions constitutes a forefront in clinical practice. What is "special" today may soon be standardized by better awareness of basic physiology and improved testing controls. The ophthalmologist is being pressured in this direction by (1) conscientious patients seeking care and advice in these functions, (2) agencies concerned with operator licensing in various forms of transportation, (3) safety experts seeking to design systems for humans based on their visual (as well as other) functions, (4) concern of insurance carriers to identify and quantitate risks, and (5) adversaries seeking to establish responsibility and negligence under law.

GLARE

Glare or dazzle is the unpleasant effect of unneeded light striking the retina and impairing vision at that time. In the early decades of this century much attention was directed to the glare component because of lens fluorescence evoked by ultraviolet light between 375 and 400 mμ. This wavelength is absorbed by the lens to a high degree in youth and almost completely after middle life; the shorter ultraviolet is absorbed almost entirely by the cornea. Lens fluorescence superimposes some blurring or fogging of the retinal image formed by visible light (400 to 700 mμ). Of greater functional significance, however, is the glare caused by excessive visible light itself.

Glare may be evaluated either on (1) the physical characteristics of the source or (2) the functional impairment it creates in acuity or comfort. The potential for glare increases with the intensity and area of the source. The intensity of glare, in common with basic laws of light, decreases proportionally to the square of its distance from the observer and directly with the cosine of the angle of incidence. Thus a glare source 1 foot away, if removed to 10 feet, delivers only one-hundredth of the light energy previously delivered. Or if a glare source is removed laterally to an angle of 60°, the incident rays lose at least 50% of their effectivity. Translated into practical terms, there is very little visual advantage gained in widening the medians of divided highways in excess of 50 feet.

Subjectively, glare is qualitatively classified into (1) veiling, (2) discomforting, (3) disabling, and (4) blinding. Intolerance to glare roughly increases with age but is also influenced by many subjective variables that make absolute quantitation on a mathematical base essentially impossible.

At low and medium intensities (below disabling or blinding glare), mathematical attempts have been made to utilize a *veiling function* or *veiling equivalent* to quantitate reductions in acuity or needed increments in target stimulus for glare tests. The Crawford-Stiles[1] "Glare-Meter" of 1935 was built on this principle, as have been many, more recent instruments.

A subsequent function designated as "glare recovery time" and approximated in seconds attempts to quantitate the interval required for an individual to regain "preglare" central acuity. In a fashion roughly similar to dark adaptation, this can be divided into an initial or alpha recovery phase, which is rapid, and a following or beta phase, which is slow. Marked individual variations occur particularly in practical, clinical approaches without photic prestressing and preadaptation as appropriate in laboratory experiments.[2] The effects of available pupillary diameter and speed of pupillary response have wide and separate functions from those of retinal sensitivity. Thus their control with drugs or artificial pupils is necessary in experimental studies separating out the responses of percipient cells in the retina. In the clinical or life situation, however, these pupillary components should be retained during attempts to assess glare tolerance or glare recovery time.

Test methods concerning glare are generally divided into (1) glare tolerance or acuity in the presence of standardized glare and (2) glare recovery time or the number of seconds required for acuity to regain a preglare level. Laboratory techniques, which are properly concerned with absolute values and minimal threshold measures, cannot be translated into simple clinical procedures. Several major adaptometers, however, are marketed, and these include testing under glare or dazzle. The Goldmann-Weekers adaptometer (1950) made by Haag-Streit of Bern, Switzerland, is one of the best known and standardized compromises between laboratory and clinical testing. It is too complex for mass screening and should be reserved for critical studies of uncertain cases.

Instruments of more restricted function and simpler in construction than the major adaptometers are the Recording Nyctometer, made by Carl Zeiss of Jena; the Aulhorn projection mesoptometer, made by Oculus Products of Tubingen, Germany; the Henkind-Siegel[3] hand-held scotometer (1967), made by Medin Corporation of Wallington, New Jersey; and the Night Sight Meter (1953), made by the American Automobile Association of Washington, D. C.

The smallest and most portable of these is the monocular scotometer devised by Henkind and Siegel. A preglare acuity reading is always made. It is based on an optically simulated distance Snellen reading card. This unit, like the larger Aulhorn mesoptometer, presents a commonly accepted 10-second duration of glare. After the glare, the patient strives to attain his preglare recognition of the reduced Snellen letters through the fading afterimage. With this instrument, normal glare recovery under age 40 should be less than 40 seconds. In age or disease, it may be prolonged to 180 seconds or more. The instrument has had extensive trial by Colonel Budd Appleton at Walter Reed Army Hospital in evaluation of possible macular damage from antimalarial drugs.

Somewhat more versatile, and space consuming ($30 \times 10 \times 7$ inches), is the table-top AAA Night Sight Meter. This instrument includes important elements of dynamic acuity measures and presents Landolt rings (C's) on a motor-driven disk at the rate of forty-five targets per minute, or angular displacement of 18 degrees per second. The patient must determine and announce one of the four possible positions (up, down, right, left) of the opening in the C every second and a half. The size of the C's simulate 20/300 acuity. Two glare sources (approximately 1 ft-c) may be presented 9 degrees to the left of the target, simulating headlights approaching on a two-lane road (20 feet wide) at a distance of 150 feet. Target illumination is then increased to the level necessary for target recognition, and this is an empirical measure of glare tolerance. To quantitate glare recovery, the glare sources are extinguished and target illumination is simultaneously reduced to the minimum level required for preglare recognition. With the aid of an interval timer, the examiner notes the seconds elapsing until the patient just regains ability to see the moving targets under his preglare conditions.

In a clinical evaluation of this instrument, Keeney and Erdbrink[4] found that 10% of a group of 162 consecutive eye patients fitted for spectacle correction in the absence of any apparent morphologic changes of pathology were unable to meet the demands of this test procedure.

DYNAMIC VISUAL ACUITY (ACUITY IN THE PRESENCE OF MOTION)

Static measurements of visual acuity have been quantitated in terms of the *minimum separable* since the mid-1700's, but study of the effects of motion on central acuity or resolving power date only from the late 1930's, and primarily from the extensive studies of Elek Ludvigh,[5] of the Kresge Eye Institute, since the mid-1940's. Discrimination of real motion or the minimum visible threshold for recognition of stimulus motion is at the fovea and is related to visual acuity. The simple appreciation of motion, however, especially in low illumination, seems best in the retinal periphery, where it is often vague, poorly localized, and subjectively exaggerated. Dynamic visual acuity seems to depend on functions in addition to those determining static visual acuity.

In-line or closing movement between target and observer obviously yields a gradient of increasing resolving power, but the effect of angular displacement impairs acuity in relation to the angular velocity. Both form recognition and resolving power decay more with observer than with target movement. This is not a linear relation but is asymptotic with a sharp increase in the rate of decay around 50 degrees per second. Some compensation occurs with increasing time of stimulus exposure up to 1 second or increasing illumination, but light levels must go up by about 3 log units to improve dynamic acuity by a factor of 2 or 3. The effects of vertical displacement parallel those of horizontal displacement but are less by a minute or two of arc in acuity measurements. Also, such displacement motions when in a straight line cause less decay than when in a circular path at identical velocities. If acceleration is added to target speed, further deterioration in acuity will result. Above 100 degrees per second visual acuity is reduced to essentially gross field blurs.

Though variations up to a factor of 10 may be obtained in dynamic acuity measurements of different individuals, even when the eyes are free of apparent pathological changes, the relationship of the components of dynamic acuity are generally unaltered. These factors may assume major importance, as among a population of flying personnel all of whom have uncorrected central acuity of 20/20 or better. Miller and Ludvigh[6] have plotted such findings in aviation cadets and found that frequency distribution histograms more nearly approximate Poisson (higher median and narrower distribution) than gaussian curves. About 90% of test subjects will show distinct improvement in dynamic acuity with practice, and about half of such improvement will be attained after three or four trials. After ten trials, most subjects will have attained more than 90% of the improvement that can be seen after twenty trials. Extended training over a few weeks has little yield.

Mechanically, as part of a servomechanism, the eyes can follow[7] accurately a moving target up to a speed of about 30 to 40 degrees per second. This is a smooth tracking movement rather than the saccadic movement commonly used to achieve or change fixation. Pursuit movements begin to disintegrate at 50 to 75 degrees per second and are completely disintegrated at 90 to 100 degrees per second. The average speed of voluntary or willed versions is between 100 and 200 degrees per second for small movements and over 500 degrees per second for large angles. This cannot be varied except by making pauses.

The impairment of acuity with movement of either the stimulus or the subject apparently relates only in small measure to extrafoveal position of the retinal image but is largely the result of physiological latencies and speed of neural transmissions creating inaccuracies or inexactness of ocular pursuit and control. Age, fatigue, tonus, and general integrity of the oculomotor system also have a role in the status of dynamic acuity.

There is little correlation between static and dynamic measurements of visual acuity, and, in a given individual, there may be a lack of correlation between acuity at low- and high-angular velocities.

In addition to the primary role of angular displacement affecting dynamic visual acuity and the secondary roles of positive and negative accelerations, there is a labyrinthine input added by head movements, nonlinear travel, or vehicular turning and maneuvering. Stimuli may thus be evoked by movements of endolymph within the semicircular canals causing reflex versional movements or nystagmus ("Coriolis effect"). This may create transient visual illusions or motion sickness.

Vibration, as a component in studies of the effect of motion, has received particular attention by research physiologists in the armed services. Generally, in all forms of land transportation as well as in helicopters and low flying aircraft, the greater the velocity of the vehicle, the greater the amplitude of vibration. Frequencies most disturbing to vision are between 25 and 40 cps. Both increasing amplitude and increasing frequency cause decay in acuity, but the rate of decrement levels off at frequencies above 60 cps.[8]

There are literally thousands of studies, emanating primarily from the field of psychology, analyzing a wide variety of geometrical factors that seem to have bearing on subjective interpretation. These include angular size, contour, sharpness of outline, horizontal versus vertical disposition, intensity, color, background, pattern, contrast, and the like.

The extensive studies by Albert Burg[9] at the University of California at Los Angeles have correlated dynamic visual acuity and other visual tests with actual records of 17,500 California drivers. His data show dynamic visual acuity to have the strongest relation of all visual tests to actual crash experience. Static visual acuity follows after a major interval as a much weaker second-level predictor.

The term "speed smear" has been used as the environmental correlation of "optical smear" or "retinal blur" to indicate reductions in acuity from relative movement between observer and target or during saccadic movements, either involuntary or associated with changes in fixation. On noting that, when gazing into a mirror, eye movements are not seen when fixation is being changed, observers from 1898 through the early 1900's felt that vision was absent during these saccades. Actually, however, a reduced level of acuity is present during voluntary and involuntary saccades, which is proportional to the speed or movement of the retinal image.[10]

Importance in this subject attaches to millions of land transport drivers (100 million licensed in the United States alone), and particularly to flying personnel* in low-level flight (involved in every takeoff and landing), as well as in helicopter operations, mapping, reconnaissance, concealed attack, and so on.

CHANGES WITH AGING

> The aging eye—like the dying Goethe—needs more light.
>
> R. A. Weale, 1963

Structural alterations in the globes

With somewhat mathematically predictable progression, there is a diffuse involutional arteriolosclerosis (of Albutt) characteristic of advancing decades and involving the entire body vasculature. It is independent of blood pressure, although its inroads may be compounded by hypertension. Its levels of retinal, choroidal, and cerebral involvement are often not parallel. It causes progressive diminution of both retinal sensitivity and cerebral cortical response.[11] These changes may have clinical manifestations and may be seen in histological sections occasionally as early as the third and fourth decade of life; they are almost universally present after the fifth or sixth decade. They may be diffuse or areolar. These changes lead to both degeneration and hyperplasia in the hyaline portion of Bruch's membrane. Some change of basophilic staining and thickening

---

*See documents of Vision Committee, Advisory Group for Aerospace Research and Development (AGARD) of the North Atlantic Treaty Organization, Paris, France.

may become evident at the age of 30. Small discrete, whitish-yellow areas of depigmentation may be seen in the retinal periphery on indirect ophthalmoscopic examination after the age of 30 or 35, and in nearly half of all individuals beyond the age of 40. These peripheral involutional changes have been described as paving stone or cobble-stone degeneration.[12]

Of associated and cumulative significance are morphological changes of age (gerontological changes) occurring in practically every ocular tissue.

Cornea. Guttate dystrophy or Hassall-Henle bodies extending into the endothelium from the level of Descemet's membrane and spreading from the periphery involve the entire cornea with advancing decades. Increasing horizontal curvature, Krukenberg spindles, and Hudson-Stahli lines are additional manifestations.

Pupils. The pupillary diameter shows progressive reduction (miosis) and commensurate light exclusion beginning in early adult years. Sphincter hyalinization and stromal rigidity also impair the potential for dilation and enhanced light admission under subdued illumination.

Anterior chamber. The anterior chamber becomes progressively shallow, predisposing to mydriatic or acute congestive glaucoma.

Lens. Throughout life, there is increasing lens thickness. This leads to progressive relucency, yellowing, and scattering (diffraction) of light within layers of the lens after adolescence. The yellowing, however, may compensate in part for reduction in macular pigment.

Vitreous. Micellar beading and atrophy lead to vitreous cavitation, posterior detachment, and collapse.

Luteal pigment (leaf xanthophil). With each decade of adult life there is darkening and absorption of luteal pigment in the yellow spectral area. In the first decades of life this reduces light scatter and increases resolving power. Its loss is accompanied by physiological reduction in macular acuity, which may be measured as a line or two on the Snellen chart. (Rarely, therefore, a patient with early involutional macular changes will attain improvement in central acuity with the aid of a yellow [Wratten K1 or K2] spectacle lens.)

Orbit. Fat atrophy and tissue dehydration lead to recession of the globe.

Functional impairments of vision with age

Although reduction in visual ability primarily derives from retinal vascular involution, there is slowing of interpretative function, which augments the total reduction in ocular effectiveness. Localization of some of these losses to the retina itself is evidenced by electroretinographic dimution in b-waves with advancing age.[13] Clinically, this is accompanied by impairments in mesopic acuity, glare tolerance, and glare recovery. Light intensities required for threshold vision increase by about 1 log unit, as threshold intensities for light sensation after dark adaptation increase by about 3 log units between the second and eighth decades of life.

The totality of changes requires virtually double the amount of illumination for equal seeing under mesopic conditions for every 13 years of adult life.[14,15] Scotopic spectral sensitivity particularly shows marked loss at short wavelengths as age advances. However, for usual photopic tasks, a local illumination increase by a factor of 2 or 3 compensates for losses between the second and sixth decades. Because of increased light scatter, especially in the lens, elderly persons will prefer yellowish to cold white or bluish light.

The youthful emmetropic eye also becomes physiologically hyperopic by a diopter or two with advancing years (a disadvantage that can be offset by modest myopia in early life). This may be counterbalanced by early cataractous change in the lens with its induced myopic shift caused by lens intumescence.

Snellen acuity as quantitated for distance decreases modestly from the sixth through later decades so that 20/25 or less central vision is expected even in the absence of gross morphological disturbances. For reasons difficult to identify and quantitate, these decrements may be modestly less in the near or reading range than under distance test conditions. Between age 80 and 90, the central acuity may drop to 20/30 or 20/40. Similarly, there is slight constriction in the visual fields. This may be exaggerated by orbital fat atrophy, creating relative enophthalmos with corresponding obscuration of the visual field in its peripheral areas.

Subtle defects in hue discrimination also creep in with advancing maturity of the eye. This commonly mimics anomalous tritanopia but is not a gross defect.

Less frequently tested functions show progressive reductions, as in critical flicker fusion frequencies, visual reaction time, speed of visual performance, and dark adaptation. Small comfort may be taken in the fact that the presbyopic patient is no longer affected by the 0.50 to 1.00D or so of night myopia or empty space myopia that affects the nonpresbyopic patient.

Common, classifiable geriatric pathology or ocular diseases in advancing years seem to increase arithmetically after the fourth decade of life. Kornzweig[16] has tabulated these population groups in a large retirement home and found some degree of cataract present in about 50% of those 60 to 80, but 75% of those over 80. Macular disease was identifiable in 20% of those from 60 to 80 and about 40% of those over 80. Glaucoma occurs in nearly 15% of patients in each decade after age 60.

Thus both the physiological inroads of chronology and a group of age-related eye diseases combine to reduce the individual's ability to maintain his earlier effectiveness in coping with the usual visual environment.

> Apart from these two conditions—lens yellowing and increased depth of focus due to miosis—however, there is little to be said in favor of senility.
>
> R. A. Weale, 1963

REFERENCES

1. Crawford, B. H., and Stiles, W. S.: A brightness difference threshold meter for the evaluation of glare from light sources, J. Sci. Instrum. **12:**177, 1935.
2. Severin, S. L., Tour, R. L., and Kershaw, R. H.: Macular function and the photostress test, Arch. Ophthal. (Chicago) **77:**163, 1967.
3. Henkind, P., and Siegel, I. M.: The scotometer, Amer. J. Ophthal. **64:**314, 1967.
4. Keeney, A. H., and Erdbrink, W. L.: Mesopic vision, glare tolerance and glare recovery, Proceedings of 10th Annual Meeting, American Association of Automotive Medicine, pp. 36-39, 1966.
5. Miller, J. W., and Ludvigh, E. J.: The effect of relative motion on visual acuity, Survey Ophthal. **7:**83, 1962.

6. Miller, J. W., and Ludvigh, E. J.: Results of testing dynamic visual acuity of 1000 naval aviation cadets, Kresge Eye Institute and U. S. Naval School of Aviation Medicine, Joint Project N.M. 001 501, Report No. 10, 1956.

7. Moses, R. A.: Adler's physiology of the eye, ed. 5, St. Louis, 1970, The C. V. Mosby Co., pp. 210, 216.

8. Drazin, D.: Factors affecting vision during vibration, Research 15:275, 1962.

9. Burg, A.: Some relationships between vision and driving, Proceedings of 11th Annual Meeting, American Association of Automotive Medicine, Springfield, Ill., 1970, Charles C Thomas, Publisher, pp. 61-69.

10. Duntley, S. Q., and others: Visibility, LaJolla, 1964, Scripps Institute of Oceanography, University of California.

11. Weale, R. A.: The aging eye, London, 1963, H. K. Lewis & Company Ltd.

12. Meyer-Schwickerath, G.: Light coagulation (translated by S. M. Drance), St. Louis, 1960, The C. V. Mosby Co.

13. Karpe, G., Rickenbach, K., and Thomassen, S.: The clinical ERG: 1, The normal ERG above 50 years of age, Acta Ophthal. 28:301, 1950.

14. McFarland, R. A., Domey, R. G., and Warren, A. B.: Night visibility: dark adaptation as a function of age and tinted windshield glass, Highway Res. Board Bull. 255:47, 1960.

15. McFarland, R. A., and others: Dark adaptation as a function of age, J. Geront. 15:149, 1960.

16. Kornzweig, A. L., Feldstein, M., and Schneider, J.: The eye in old age, Amer. J. Ophthal. 44:29, 1957.

Index

A

Abeta-lipoproteinemia, 96
Abney effect, 113-114
Abnormal color vision, 136-154
Abnormalities
  of dark-adaptation time, 92-93
  of night vision, 86-91
  progressive, of dark-adaptation thresholds, 95-98
  stationary, of final threshold, 93-98
Absolute intensity threshold, 12
Absolute threshold to light, 37
Absorption
  quantum, 65
  rhodopsin, of light quanta, 66
Absorption difference spectra, 128
Absorption spectrum, 66
AC/A ratio, 85
Accommodation, 38
Accommodative convergence to accommodation (AC/A) ratio, 85
Achromatopsia
  with amblyopia, 146-148
  without amblyopia, 148-149
Acid-N-retinylidene-opsin complex, 63
Acquired color vision defects, 152-154
  groups of, 153-154
Activation, lateral, and lateral inhibition, 51-54
Acuity(ies), 3, 4, 5, 9
  bases of, 12-23
  in presence of motion, 209-211
  resolution, 6-8
  shape-detection, 9
  Snellen, 3, 213
  spatial, 9-12
  stereoscopic, 165
  vernier, 9-10
  visibility, 5-6
  visual; see Visual acuity
Adaptation, 189
  dark; see Dark adaptation
  light, 78
  neural, 81
  state of, 40
  theory of, 79-81
  visual, 57-102

Adapting luminance, 40
Adaptometer
  continuous recording, 70
  Goldmann-Weekers, 71-72, 86-87, 208
  McLaughlin, 69, 72
Additive and subtractive mixtures, 111
  using filters, 110
Aerial perspective, 171
After-image, 80-81, 129
Age, functional impairments of vision with, 212-213
Aging, changes with, 211-213
Algebra of color mixture, 121-122
All-trans retinal, 63, 66
Alteration(s)
  in dark-adaptation curve, 76
  structural, in globes, 211-212
Amaurosis, congenital, of Leber, 195
Amblyopia
  achromatopsia with, 146-148
  achromatopsia without, 148-149
  hysterical, 98
Ametropic blur, effect of, 37-38
Amplifier, 190
Analysis, Granit, of electroretinogram, 193-194
Anatomical sites for electrophysiological measurements, 203
Angle, parallactic, 164
Anomaloscope, 145
  Nagel, 145, 146, 147, 153
Anomalous trichromatism, 151-152
Anterior chamber, 212
Apparatus
  for measuring dark-adaptation curve, 69-72
  for recording visual evoked response, 198
  rotating plane, 176
    settings of, 176, 177
Appearance, color, 111-114
Applications, clinical, of electro-oculogram, 201-203
Arago's phenomenon, 60
Area
  Panum's, 163, 164, 165, 168
  Piper's, 37
  Ricco's, 37
Armed Forces National Research Council Vision Committee, 86

215